SOBRIETY WORKBOOK FOR WOMEN

SOBRIETY WORKBOOK for WOMEN

Practical Strategies to Live and Thrive without Alcohol

Jennifer Leupp, LCSW

ROCKRIDGE
PRESS

Interior and Cover Designer: Regina Stadnik
Art Producer: Samantha Ulban
Editor: John Makowski
Production Manager: Martin Worthington

Illustrations © Creative Market/Venimo
author photo courtesy of Zencare

Paperback ISBN: 978-1-63878-297-1
    eBook ISBN: 978-1-63878-501-9
R0

I'd like to dedicate this book to all the people in the recovery communities who helped me get sober and stay sober, and to my yoga instructors who taught me skills that have supported me emotionally.

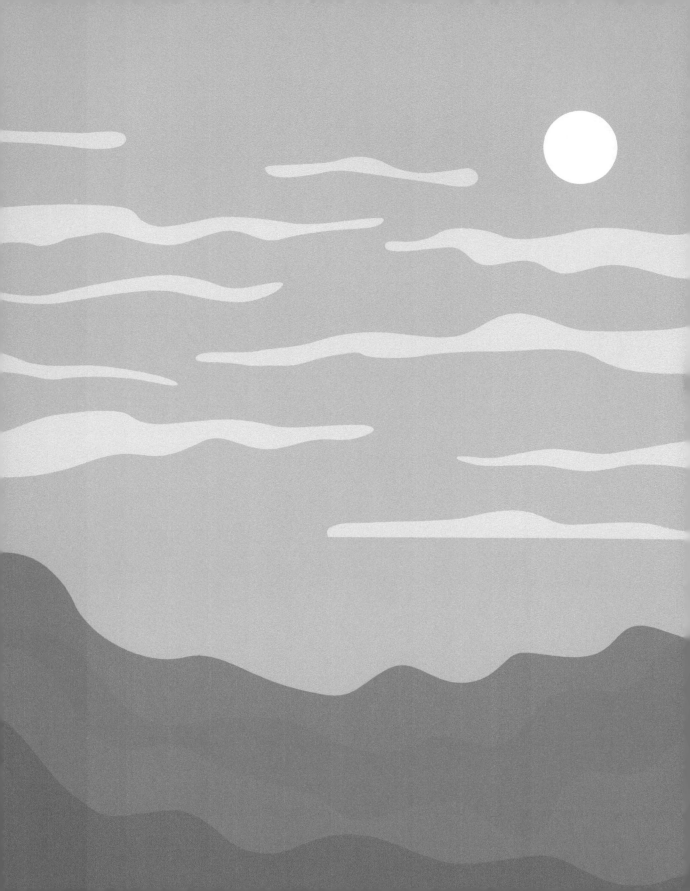

CONTENTS

INTRODUCTION

Hello! I'm Jennifer Leupp, a licensed clinical social worker (LCSW) in California with a master's degree in social work from California State University at Dominguez Hills. In my private psychotherapy practice, I specialize in working with substance abuse, relationship issues, and trauma. For the first couple years of my career, I provided psychotherapy at an inpatient drug and alcohol rehabilitation center. I also have personal experience with recovery from alcohol addiction, having received support from 12-step and Buddhist recovery communities as well as yoga and meditation communities. Through my continued use of these tools and support systems, I have found a much better life! And I believe you can, too.

If you are reading this book, it is likely that you either want to reduce or abstain from alcohol or help someone else who wants to do so. Making the decision to change your relationship with alcohol is no small feat. It requires lifestyle changes, learning new skills and tools to support yourself emotionally, and letting go of some relationships and creating new ones. Most importantly, it includes changing your relationship with yourself. It takes courage to embark on such a journey, and I commend you on taking this first step.

In recent years there has been a drastic increase in drinking and alcohol dependency among women. I believe that tailoring a workbook specifically for women who want to quit drinking is essential because there are particular issues women are uniquely impacted by that many other recovery books and programs fail to address. These issues include the ways in which we are marketed to, the ways that alcohol affects our bodies and our emotions, and the gender-specific ways we are taught to deal (or not deal) with our feelings. As a woman, I am inspired and honored by this opportunity to address other women in the hope that my knowledge and experience can support them.

This book is meant to assist individuals who want to find a healthy and sustainable way to get sober by treating the underlying issues and pressures that drive them to drink. Many of us have found some recovery communities to feel judgmental, noninclusive, or downright unsafe for women, so I wanted to provide a nonjudgmental, open, and safe space for women to explore their issues with alcohol. There is more than one way to heal and recover from alcoholism, and some approaches don't work for everyone. That is why it is important to have a variety of tools, skills, and knowledge under your belt to support you in your recovery. I hope this book can help you do just that.

Congratulations on seeking help! I encourage you to work through this workbook thoroughly to help guide and support you in your recovery, because with each step you take, you are moving toward reclaiming your life. The work may seem challenging or daunting at times, but it's definitely worth it—your hard work will soon show you the freedom, wholeness, and happiness that can be found as you move forward on this journey!

HOW TO USE THIS BOOK

This workbook provides you with research-based information, personal anecdotes, and client experience; exercises to help you understand the concepts; and periodic self check-ins to help you become aware of your emotions and be kind to yourself. The reading portions of this workbook provide a foundation of knowledge that explains alcoholism and the alcohol industry, emphasizing that alcohol dependence is about more than just having too much to drink. In order to heal from alcoholism in a culture that is obsessed with it, you must have a better, clear understanding of your triggers and what's causing you to drink.

Everyone's sobriety journey is different. Many readers will come to understand that complete abstinence from alcohol is the best decision for their long-term health. Healing for some may not mean entirely eliminating drinking but rather a reduction in alcohol consumption and an increase in self-awareness. Regardless of your particular path to clarity, you will be acquiring tools and strategies that will help you address underlying issues and manage strong emotions that have led to drinking as a form of escape in the past.

It is important to note that this book is not meant to replace therapy or medical advice. Many readers will find that working with a therapeutic professional or becoming a part of a recovery community is a necessary part of their sobriety journey. In order to make the most out of this book, read through each chapter, one at a time, and complete the exercises to the best of your ability. It may be helpful to set aside a time during the week or during the day and mark your calendar with that time, setting reminders if necessary. Find a quiet, calm, and comfortable place to read the book and complete the exercises. Aim to read at least one chapter each week and incorporate the exercises that you find most helpful into your daily life.

PART 1

UNDERSTANDING SOBRIETY

I am open to reflecting on my relationship with alcohol. I am open to learning new tools that will support me in developing the relationship that I would like to have with alcohol.

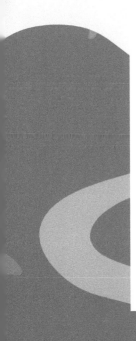

Chapter 1

MORE THAN
JUST ALCOHOL

In this chapter, we will explore the reasons why women drink and complete writing exercises to help us understand our relationship to alcohol. We will discuss our society's obsession with alcohol, identify what alcohol dependence is and is not, and contemplate what the process of asking for help has been like for us. We will review the science of alcohol and the risk factors for alcoholism and complete a self-assessment to determine our relationship to alcohol.

WHY WOMEN DRINK

Alcohol has been normalized and integrated into many aspects of our society and into many facets of our lives. We drink to celebrate, we drink when we are looking for some relief after work, we drink when we are meeting up with colleagues, we drink to soothe our nerves in social situations, we drink at sporting events, we drink to pledge our loyalty to social groups in college, we drink to fit in at parties in high school, we drink at family dinners and on dates. The list of social events at which it is expected to consume alcohol goes on and on.

Advertisements for alcohol have been increasingly targeted at women in recent years.

Ads that are marketed toward women often emphasize relationships and feeling states that women are seeking, such as empowerment, relaxation, sexiness, and friendship. From "chick beer" to "mummy's time-out" to "wine time," advertisements are making their way into many women's brains in a not-so-subtle way. Women are constantly bombarded with the messaging that alcohol can be used to de-stress, to relax, to loosen up, to provide social lubrication, and to have casual sex and connect with others. If you find that you are drinking more than you would like to, it's perfectly understandable how you got to this point.

Below are just a few reasons why women drink.

Because of a Desire to Fit In (Peer Pressure)

As adults, the idea of being peer pressured may seem unlikely, but if we consider the prevalence of people-pleasing tendencies, particularly among women, this concept makes more sense. Even though you are intent on quitting drinking, you might feel pressured to drink because it feels weird or impolite to not drink when a friend is drinking. This is an example of how people-pleasing behaviors can sometimes lead to us acquiescing to peer pressure, because many of us who have these tendencies want to make other people feel better at the expense of our own desires, needs, and feelings.

Because We Want to (Desire)

For many of us, put quite simply, we drink because we want to. We may want to drink to celebrate success, mark the end of a long workday, or have fun and let loose at a social event, or just because it feels good and provides pleasure. Social drinking is often expected in our culture on dates and at parties, clubs, sporting events, and music events. Due to marketing and social norms, drinking also often carries with it a "coolness" factor many women may be unconscious of that impacts our desire to drink.

Because We Feel Compelled to (Emotional Management)

Many of us feel compelled to drink in order to manage our emotions. We may have had a particularly rough day at work or had an anger-fueled argument with a loved one, or we may want to drink to reduce anxiety, stress, or depression. Alcohol can seem effective in coping with emotions; however, it is a short-term solution that can result in long-term consequences. Many of us aren't taught healthy emotional regulation and coping skills as children, or we experienced trauma and learned that alcohol made the pain go away.

Because We Don't Have Anything Else to Do (Boredom)

Some of us drink out of habit, because we feel we don't have anything better to do, or because there is a lack of passion or excitement in our lives. Boredom can lead many alcoholics to relapse and consume excessive amounts of alcohol even when they have a sobriety goal. Some of the clients that I have worked with have identified boredom as one of the many reasons why they have relapsed in the past. For many women struggling with overconsumption of alcohol, maintaining an active, fulfilling life can be pertinent to staying sober or drinking less.

EXPLORE YOUR TRIGGERS

Take a moment to reflect on the last time that you drank. What was going on for you that made you want to drink? What emotions were you feeling and how did you want to feel after drinking? Was your desire for alcohol related to any of the reasons why many of us drink, such as emotional regulation, personal desire, peer pressure, or boredom? Make a note of the reasons why you drank and then see if you can come up with any other ways in which you may be able to achieve a similar emotional outcome.

_____

_____

_____

_____

_____

_____

OUR OBSESSION WITH ALCOHOL

Alcohol is everywhere in our society. It's in advertisements, in movies and television shows, and at social gatherings, music shows, sports games, family events, parties, dance clubs, casinos, weddings, and more. We receive the messaging that "everybody" drinks, and often to excess—not just people with low self-esteem and self-control. The 2019 National Survey on Drug Use and Health (NSDUH) cites that approximately 55 percent of people over the age of 18 had an alcoholic beverage in the last month, and 51 percent of those individuals were women.

External factors like marketing, social interactions, and socioeconomic pressures play a significant role in why alcohol is so prevalent in our culture. Social learning theory tells us that people tend to be influenced by what they view in the media (commercials, magazines, TV, movies, and social media) and by what they observe among family and friends. Therefore, multiple avenues are available to marketers of alcohol to sell their product. As the world of advertising has grown and become more and more savvy, alcohol consumption has increased as well. In fact, a 2019 global study published in *The Lancet* determined that alcohol consumption has increased 70 percent over the last 30 years.

Marketing

With women's socioeconomic power rising in recent years, so has the marketing of alcohol toward women. Smart people have figured out how to target advertising right where women are most vulnerable, promising that their products will help us let loose, forget about our responsibilities for the moment, connect with our friends, and increase our sex appeal.

In addition to direct advertising like TV commercials and print ads, much of this marketing is often subtle, even subconscious. For instance, music has been increasingly used as a vehicle for marketing alcohol in the past couple of decades. According to a 2013 study published in *Substance Use & Misuse*, almost a quarter of the songs on Billboard's Hot 100 chart between 2009 and 2011 included mentions of alcohol.

Social Interactions

In our society, alcohol is often the centerpiece of social interactions. From the quintessential "boozy brunch" and holiday celebrations to parties, clubs, and sporting games, alcohol is used as a social lubricant, a tool of celebration, and a way to bond with friends and family, cultivating a sense of belonging and identity. Many people who have social anxiety or self-esteem challenges may depend on alcohol to help them get through events like dates, work functions, or celebratory gatherings. Learning to separate social interactions from alcohol consumption can be challenging for many of us, yet this separation plays an important role in maintaining sobriety.

Socioeconomic Escape

For many of us, alcohol assists us in temporarily escaping our less than ideal socioeconomic situations. We may kick back with a few drinks after long hours at multiple jobs in order to make the divide between work and relaxation more obvious. We may drink to forget that we are unhappy with our current financial, housing, or transportation situation. We may also drink in order to cope with the difficult feelings that come along with being marginalized.

What Drinking Is Not

Understanding what triggers us to want to drink can help us gain more self-awareness, which can then lead us to find alternative solutions to our triggers. For instance, we may not be aware that we tend to drink when we feel anxious or insecure, or when we have relationship or work problems. Once we become aware of our triggers, we can brainstorm healthier ways to cope such as utilizing meditation, thought reframing, communicating effectively, and setting healthy boundaries.

Oftentimes, people who have a problem with drinking beat themselves up for past behaviors or actions. Being trapped in this cycle of shame can keep them from truly accepting they have a problem and responding wisely to it. Because drinking is so socially accepted in our society and ingrained into a variety of aspects of our culture, it can be challenging for us to recognize that we do have a problem. It may be particularly difficult when excessive drinking is normal in our family and friend groups. Accepting that we have a drinking problem as well as accepting past behaviors can help us move on, love, and forgive ourselves, and reach our goal of sobriety or reducing drinking.

Gaining an awareness of what constitutes "problem drinking" can help us become more aware and accepting of ourselves. It is likewise helpful to be clear that problem drinking is *not*:

✳ only about alcohol

✳ equivalent to weakness

✳ a sign that you are a bad person

✳ something you have to live with forever

Being aware of what problem drinking is not can help us gain a deeper understanding of what leads us to drink, can reduce shame that we feel due to our drinking, and can provide us with hope for the future to know that change is possible.

REFLECTION ON ASKING FOR HELP

Many people struggle with asking for help, especially those struggling with alcohol misuse. What do you think kept you from asking for help until now? What was it that finally motivated you to seek help?

_____

_____

_____

_____

Being dependent on alcohol can often impact our lives in a variety of negative ways. Some alcohol dependents get into legal trouble, such as receiving DUIs, getting into domestic violence disputes, or going to jail. Some alcoholics experience employment, family, or health-related issues. How do you think dependence on alcohol has impacted your life thus far?

_____

_____

_____

_____

Identifying what we would like to change about our lives can help us have a vision for our future and create a mold for what we want. Going forward, what would you like to change about your drinking habits and about your life in general?

_____

_____

_____

_____

SCIENCE OF ALCOHOL

Alcohol, otherwise known as ethanol, is the ingredient found in liquor, wine, and beer that causes intoxication. Excessive short- and long-term consumption of alcohol has been shown to have negative health effects on the brain and the body. Even one time of excessive alcohol consumption can cause long-term health effects and death.

So, what exactly does alcohol do to the brain and body? Alcohol has been shown to have negative health effects on the brain, heart, liver, and pancreas, and is linked to certain types of cancer and a weaker immune system. Alcohol is most frequently processed by two enzymes that help separate the alcohol molecule and remove it from the body. Initially, alcohol dehydrogenase (ADH) breaks down alcohol into acetaldehyde, a carcinogenic and extremely toxic substance. Next, the ADH is transformed into acetate, after which it is metabolized into carbon dioxide and water in order to remove it from the body.

Alcohol and the Brain

Recent studies of alcoholism published by the National Institute on Alcohol Abuse and Alcoholism have shown that multiple neurotransmitters are involved in the development of alcohol dependence. In particular, it is the imbalance of various neurotransmitters in the brain that has been connected with alcohol dependence. Studies show that long-term use has also been linked to mental health conditions such as anxiety and depression. Additionally, chronic alcohol use has been linked to memory and learning problems, which can lead to poor school performance and dementia, as well as psychosis, self-harm, and suicide.

Long-term, heavy alcohol consumption may result in brain deficits that continue even after extended periods of sobriety. Heavy drinking may also negatively impact memory and could potentially lead to conditions that impair the ability to take care of oneself.

Alcohol and the Body

Long-term, excessive consumption of alcohol has been linked to the development of chronic illnesses and severe health issues such as heart disease, high blood pressure, liver disease, stroke, and digestive issues. Cancer has also been linked to excessive alcohol consumption, especially cancer of the throat, mouth, breast, voice box, esophagus, colon, rectum, and liver.

Alcohol has also been shown to weaken the immune system, which can make it more likely that you will develop an illness such as tuberculosis or pneumonia. A weakened immune system also makes it more difficult for the body to resist infections.

RISK FACTORS FOR ALCOHOLISM

Historically, alcoholism has most often been associated with men, but women (of all ages) have increasingly been closing the gender gap in alcohol consumption and misuse. In fact, recent data from the Substance Abuse and Mental Health Services Administration and researchers at Michigan University's Institute for Social Research shows that women in their teens and 20s reported drinking and getting drunk at even higher rates than their male peers. Many individuals often develop problems with drinking in their teens and early 20s, but alcohol dependence can also develop later in life. Certain factors such as family history, mental health disorders, a history of trauma, peer pressure, and stress can increase the risk of developing a dependency on alcohol. In contrast, some of the positive effects of maintaining sobriety are improved mental health, increased self-confidence, learning to set healthy internal and external boundaries, reduced stress, improved physical health, and higher rates of success when it comes to career and relationships.

Family History

Family history plays a significant role in the risk of developing alcohol dependence. Studies on families and twins conclude that if an individual has an alcoholic family member, the risk of them becoming alcohol dependent themselves is 40 to 60 percent. This statistic does not necessarily account for the risk involved in being raised by or in the same household as an alcoholic family member. Both nature (genetics) and nurture (external factors after birth) play a significant part in the risk of an individual developing a problem with drinking.

Other Mental Health Disorders

Mental health disorders such as anxiety, depression, bipolar disorder, post-traumatic stress disorder (PTSD), and many others can also play a large role in whether an individual will develop a drinking problem. Many people use alcohol to self-medicate mental health symptoms. Although alcohol is often used to alleviate difficult emotions and mental health symptoms, maintaining sobriety can actually increase mental well-being over time. In the process of recovery, many people get into therapy or join recovery programs where they learn healthy tools to cope with mental health symptoms. Confidence is also often boosted the longer an individual is able to maintain sobriety.

Peer Pressure

Peer pressure can also present as a risk factor for developing a drinking problem. In high school and sometimes as early as middle school, many teens are under the impression that the "cool" kids drink, or that "everybody's doing it." In college, many people feel pressured to pledge to their sororities or fraternities by drinking large quantities of alcohol in a short period of time. Most colleges have a high rate of alcohol abuse on and off campus, and people may feel pressured to drink in order to fit in with their peers, to ease social anxiety, or to engage in sexual activity. As adults, we are often pressured by the same desires to fit in, which in many cases can lead to consuming excess alcohol.

Stress

Stress is another important risk factor in the potential development of an alcohol problem. Many of us drink to alleviate our stress and calm down at the end of a work day, or to deal with a downswing of a difficult relationship, or to mark the end of an intense week of school deadlines. Many of my clients have cited stress as a reason for their continued drinking or relapses. The good news is that we can learn to take care of our stress in more sustainable and healthy ways that do not cause all of the problems that alcohol can. Some ways that we can address stress are through exercise, breathing exercises, yoga, meditation, cognitive behavioral techniques, and affirmations.

SELF-ASSESSMENT: MY RELATIONSHIP WITH ALCOHOL

Evaluating your relationship with alcohol can help you gain clarity and understand whether the relationship is problematic. The following assessment will assist you in determining what the nature of your relationship is to alcohol, what your drinking patterns are, and what behaviors or habits often characterize an unhealthy relationship with alcohol. As you are completing this workbook, you may find it helpful to come back to this assessment in order to gauge your level of progress.

In the past year, have you . . .

1. Drank more or for a longer period of time than you meant to?

2. Tried to reduce or abstain from drinking but were unable to?

3. Spent substantial amounts of time drinking or became ill or found yourself recovering from the effects of alcohol?

4. Found yourself craving a drink so badly that you were not able to think of other things?

5. Found that your drinking was causing difficulties with friends and family but kept drinking anyway?

6. Drank instead of engaging in activities that you previously enjoyed?

7. Found yourself in risky situations like having unprotected sex, driving or swimming drunk, spending time in unsafe areas, or using machinery while inebriated?

8. Kept drinking after experiencing blackout episodes or after you noticed you were feeling anxious, depressed, or experiencing another health condition from drinking?

9. Noticed an increased tolerance to alcohol? (In other words, you need to drink more to get a similar effect?)

10. Experienced withdrawal symptoms like nausea, sweating, a rapid heart rate, shakiness, restlessness, trouble sleeping, hearing or seeing things that are not present, or a seizure?

According to the *Diagnostic and Statistical Manual of Mental Disorders* (*DSM-5*), if you answered yes to two of these questions, you may have alcohol use disorder (AUD). Experiencing two or three of these symptoms is indicative of mild AUD, whereas experiencing four to five of these symptoms is associated with moderate AUD. The presence of six or more of these symptoms represents severe AUD.

IT CAN GET BETTER

You may have been living with alcoholism for so long that you cannot remember what life was like when you were not struggling with this cycle. Therefore, it may be tough for you to imagine living a different life, free from the grasp of alcohol. There are countless people who have been where you are and were able to make a change. It is possible!

You are not defined by your relationship with alcohol or who you are when you drink. Although it may seem daunting, you can embrace a different lifestyle and improve your well-being.

If you read and work through this book, you are bound to notice some improvement in your relationship with alcohol, as well as your relationships with yourself and your loved ones. You don't have to do this on your own. There are a multitude of tools and resources available to you to support you in maintaining your sobriety. It's just a matter of being open and willing to try new things, finding what works for you, and committing to it.

DEBRIEF AND DIGEST

In this chapter, we covered five key lessons:

- Women drink due to a desire to fit in, because we want to, for emotional management, and out of boredom.
- We are impacted by marketing and our society's obsession with alcohol. Social interactions are often alcohol-centered, and drinking is sometimes perceived as a way to escape socioeconomic circumstances.
- Alcohol dependence is not just about alcohol, not equivalent to weakness, not a sign that you are a bad person, or not something you have to live with forever.

- Alcohol impacts the brain and body, and there are several risk factors for alcoholism, such as family history, other mental health disorders, peer pressure, and stress.
- Your life can get better through openness, willingness, and commitment.

SELF CHECK-IN

Take a moment to check in with yourself. How are you feeling after taking in this information and completing the exercises in chapter 1? Are you feeling surprised, scared, alarmed, or apprehensive? Do you feel motivated to make some changes?

Take a moment to reflect on what you have read. Did you learn anything that you were not aware of before? Did you learn anything about yourself?

I am not my emotions.
I can observe my emotions.
Noticing the physical
sensations that come
along with emotions will
help me gain awareness
and reach my goals.

Chapter 2

IN YOUR BODY

Many people are able to identify some of the emotions that they are feeling. However, the ability to connect emotions to the physical sensations we feel in our bodies can be more challenging. For instance, how would you describe the physical feeling of anger? What's its temperature? Where do you feel it in your body? Reconnecting with your body in this way is a useful tool that can help you gain the awareness that will help you get out of the cycle of drinking.

WHEN EMOTIONS FLOOD YOUR BODY

Emotions that tend to be uncomfortable for people, such as fear, guilt, anger, depression, and anxiety, are often products of our thoughts, which also manifest as physical sensations. When our bodies respond with strong physical reactions, it's hard to remember that our thoughts are just that—thoughts—and that they are not always true.

In addition, people who are dependent on alcohol may experience physical symptoms directly related to their alcohol use. It is common for people who have consumed an excessive amount of alcohol to experience physical symptoms the morning after, also known as a hangover. Some people experience alcohol withdrawal before they have had a drink for the day. There are many physical symptoms common to alcoholic episodes as well, especially if a person has consumed three or more drinks. The following is a list of physical symptoms that may arise before, during, and after an alcoholic episode.

Headaches: Many people experience a headache the morning after overconsuming alcohol, which is one of many symptoms of a hangover. People who are physically dependent on alcohol may also experience headaches when they have not yet had a drink for the day.

Lightheadedness: Lightheadedness is a common symptom that people experience when they have consumed a moderate amount of alcohol. The lightheadedness occurs when the nervous system is impaired, which also compromises coordination and slows reaction time. Lightheadedness can lead to losing consciousness if an individual continues to drink.

Difficulty breathing: Difficulty breathing is one of the symptoms of potential alcohol overdose that can lead to brain damage or death. People who experience difficulty breathing while they are drunk may also experience other warning signs of potential alcohol overdose, including extremely low temperature, mental confusion, and difficulty remaining conscious.

Chest Pain: Research shows that small amounts of alcohol may be heart healthy. However, there is also evidence that alcohol can cause heart complications. Chest pains, which are often experienced during hangovers or during withdrawal, could be indicative of angina (reduced blood flow to the heart), heart attack, or alcoholic cardiomyopathy.

Sweating: It's common to experience sweating the day after a night of excessive alcohol consumption. Alcohol can cause you to sweat because it frequently raises blood pressure and widens blood vessels. Night sweats are often experienced by those who are in withdrawal from alcohol.

Joint pain: People who drink in excess tend to experience increased levels of joint pain. Research shows that excess alcohol consumption may be linked to the development of osteoarthritis. In addition, according to the Centers for Disease Control and Prevention (CDC), the more alcohol that one consumes, the more likely they are to develop gout, a form of inflammatory arthritis.

Fatigue: After an alcoholic episode, many people experience fatigue. Increased urination and loss of fluids is often a result of alcohol consumption that can cause mild dehydration, leading to fatigue, thirst, and a headache. It is common for people who drink in excess to also experience disrupted sleep, including sleep apnea, which can cause additional fatigue.

Thirst: It's important to stay hydrated by drinking a lot of water during and after an episode of drinking. Many people who consume excess alcohol also experience increased levels of thirst the day following an alcoholic episode due to dehydration.

Nausea/stomach discomfort: Consuming alcohol causes the stomach to create additional acid, which can result in gastritis, causing the lining of the stomach to become inflamed. Gastritis leads to pain in the stomach, diarrhea, vomiting, and sometimes bleeding for those who drink heavily. Overconsumption of alcohol can also cause acid reflux and peptic ulcers.

EXPLORE PHYSICAL SYMPTOMS

Take a moment to recall and write down any recent bodily symptoms you may have experienced before, during, and after drinking excessively. What did your body feel like? Did you experience any of these physical symptoms?

_____

_____

_____

_____

The Mind-Body Connection

Over the last few decades, there has been a growing body of evidence supporting the connection between the mind and the body. Research by Jill Littrell, PhD, LCSW, has shown that stressful emotions change the way that white blood cells operate. Stress has been shown to increase the risk of viral infections and cancer due to the way it compromises the response of white blood cells. In addition, wounds have been shown to heal slower and vaccines tend to respond less effectively in individuals who are stressed. According to the research, the recurring, long-term stress that poverty causes can also weaken the immune system. Autoimmune conditions have been shown to be negatively impacted by stress as well.

The good news is that evidence has shown that talk therapy can strengthen the immune system, supporting the body's resistance to disease. In addition, mindfulness practices have been linked to reduced risk of heart disease and cell aging, a possible decrease in Alzheimer's symptoms and cancer biomarkers, and an improved immune system. Mindfulness practices can also reduce psychological pain associated with conditions like depression and anxiety, which can have a positive impact on a variety of chronic illnesses.

MINDFUL MOVEMENT

Take a moment to observe how you feel emotionally and physically. Then stand with your feet hip distance apart and your arms by your sides. Slowly and mindfully begin to extend your arms out and up toward the sky as you inhale. At the top, put your hands together in a prayer position and mindfully bring your hands down to your chest as you exhale. Repeat this 3 to 10 times. Then take a moment to observe how you feel now. Has anything changed for you, emotionally or physically? Return to this exercise as often as you'd like whenever you need to feel more centered and grounded.

CULTIVATE BODY AWARENESS

Many of us spend most of our time with our attention focused on our external world, like when we are at work or school or when we are having a conversation, scrolling social media, viewing TV/movies or videos, and reading. Because we are so accustomed to focusing on our external world, bringing attention to our internal world can often be quite challenging. For some, it can even feel scary.

When we pay attention to our internal world, we can learn to communicate with ourselves in a way that can change our emotional landscape. For instance, if we are feeling angry, we can pay attention to where we feel that in the body, focus on it, and breathe into that space, allowing our breath to cascade over those feelings. Bringing focus and breath to the sensations in our bodies can help alleviate our uncomfortable emotional responses. Cultivating body awareness and communicating with ourselves in this kind and gentle way includes the following benefits.

Quiets your mind: Mindfulness instructors often refer to our minds as "monkey minds" because we tend to jump from one thought to another, like a monkey jumps from one tree branch to another. Mindfulness practices such as yoga, meditation, and qigong can help us quiet the mind by bringing our focus to the breath, the body, a visualization, or a mantra.

Helps you learn about your body's unique response to stress/anxiety: Some of us may notice that our breath becomes more short or choppy in times of stress, whereas others may notice some tension in the throat or in the belly. Learning what your body's unique response to anxiety and stress is can help you identify and manage your emotions earlier when they are happening.

Shows you where you are most tense: Once you have identified which areas of your body hold the most tension, you can engage in physical self-care activities such as yoga, walking, Pilates, or massage to help alleviate the tension. Working on posture and cultivating an ideal ergonomic work setup can also provide some assistance with relieving tension.

Cultivates self-compassion for your body and its cues: Cultivating self-compassion is one of the key factors in maintaining sobriety. Not only can we learn to cultivate self-compassion for our pasts and our emotions but cultivating self-compassion for our bodies and their cues can make our internal world feel safer and less intimidating.

BREAKING AUTOPILOT

Many of us operate on autopilot. We may work at a computer all day and rarely check in with our emotions and how our bodies are feeling, which can result in us feeling stressed or anxious or having sore arms or a kink in our neck at the end of the day. We may run from errand to errand, finding ourselves exhausted and depleted when our to-do list is completed. Increasing awareness of your body can help interrupt your tendency to operate on autopilot and help you become more mindful of how you use your energy.

Uncomfortable emotions often have a way of forcing our bodies to turn to autopilot to function. When we're stressed, we often return to what is familiar, even if it doesn't really serve us in the end—such as drinking alcohol. Reconnecting with our bodies can help break that habit.

In what ways do you operate on autopilot in your life? When you wake up, do you immediately check your phone and social media accounts or go get breakfast ready for the family before checking in with your body or your emotions? Do you notice yourself absentmindedly reaching for a drink after work or at a social event without a second thought?

Throughout the day, when you find that you have been engaging in an activity without awareness, try taking a moment to be still. Put away anything you are working on, close your eyes, and observe what is going on in your body. Breathe. Notice what your body is telling you. What sensations are you experiencing?

DEBRIEF AND DIGEST

In this chapter, we covered five key lessons:

- Uncomfortable emotions often manifest as physical reactions in the body.
- You can reconnect with your body through mindfulness activities.
- Gaining awareness of your body can help take you out of the cycle of drinking.
- Some physical symptoms that come up before, during, and after an alcoholic episode often include lightheadedness, headaches, difficulty breathing, chest pain, thirst, and fatigue.
- Using mindfulness to bring your body out of autopilot can help reduce stress and stress-related drinking.

SELF CHECK-IN

Take a moment to check in with your emotions. How would you describe what you're feeling? Remember to breathe and notice where you are feeling your emotions in your body. Are they concentrated in one particular area? Do they have a temperature, color, or texture? Describe the sensation.

Now, take a moment to reflect on what you read in this chapter. Did you learn anything new or different? Was there anything that you could relate to or that you found helpful?

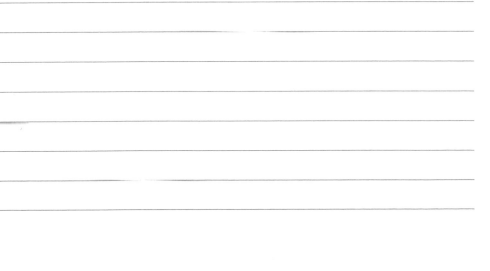

I am not my thoughts.

I can observe my thoughts.

When I observe my thoughts,

I can separate myself from

them and gain more control

over my emotions.

Chapter 3

IN YOUR BRAIN

In chapter 2 we focused on some of the physical aspects of drinking and how gaining awareness of the ways our emotions show up in our bodies can help us maintain sobriety. In this chapter, we will discuss the role that your brain plays in drinking and the thoughts and impulses that can lead to excessive drinking. The ability to gain awareness of your thoughts will help you stay away from drinking.

YOUR BRAIN ON ALCOHOL

Consuming excess alcohol significantly impacts your brain and its function. This detrimental impact can eventually lead to alcohol dependence, based on factors such as how much and how often you consume alcohol.

What occurs in our brains when we drink? Some of our brain's neurotransmitters, such as dopamine and serotonin, are highly impacted by drinking, playing an important role in what makes us feel good when drinking, what causes us to become intoxicated, what leads us back to drinking, and what ultimately can cause us to become dependent on alcohol.

When drinking provides us with pleasure or helps us avoid pain, our brains receive positive reinforcement for drinking, and we are motivated to continue or repeat the behavior. This is how the craving for alcohol develops, even when we know it's bad for us. This habitual behavior creates new neuropathways in the brain, deepening our dependence on alcohol. In the following sections we will discuss how this can play a role in drinking and the release of dopamine and serotonin.

Dopamine: What It Does and the Role It Plays

Dopamine is a neurotransmitter in the brain that transports chemicals between neurons. Often referred to as the "feel-good" neurotransmitter, dopamine is also associated with a variety of other functions such as our moods, how we make decisions, our mental health conditions, and even our motor functioning and movement.

Dopamine is connected to our sense of pleasure and reward. In fact, in times when we are expecting some type of "reward," such as sex, food, shopping, or alcohol, dopamine is released in the brain. The more your brain learns to associate alcohol with reward and these surges of dopamine, the more ingrained habitual drinking will become.

Serotonin: What It Does and the Role It Plays

Another significant neurotransmitter is serotonin, which relays information between nerve cells. Serotonin is a powerful brain chemical that stabilizes mood, regulates bowel movements and sleep, helps blood clots form, stimulates nausea, assists digestion, and impacts bone health and sexual function. Research shows that the actions that serotonin takes are also connected to the effect of alcohol on the brain and alcohol dependence. Low serotonin levels in the brain have been linked to alcoholism, and it is likely that neurotransmitters such as serotonin are linked to the inebriating and rewarding effects of alcohol. Serotonin is also thought to contribute to the effects of long-term or chronic abuse, such as increased tolerance and withdrawal symptoms like anxiety.

ADDICTION, DESIRE, AND CRAVINGS

Regions of the brain responsible for memory, pleasure, and reward play an impactful role in alcohol cravings. Various neurotransmitters such as dopamine and serotonin have been implicated in alcohol addiction due to the imbalance that alcohol causes in the brain, which could be due to either their excess activity or inhibition.

Excess alcohol consumption has been linked to difficulties when it comes to hormones, emotions, and the initial detox process. People who consume excess alcohol often experience hormonal complications that can result in a variety of physiological and behavioral issues. In addition to hormones, emotions can be negatively impacted by alcohol. Many people often self-medicate with alcohol to cope with their emotions in the short term, but they may not realize that alcohol consumption can actually increase depression, anxiety, and stress over time. The initial detox from alcohol for a person who consumes large quantities regularly can oftentimes result in withdrawal symptoms. Detoxing from alcohol can be dangerous and may need to be medically monitored, depending on the severity of alcohol dependence.

Hormones

The hormones in the body, released into the bloodstream as part of the endocrine system, control all of our biological functions throughout our lives. The reproductive system, the brain and nervous system, blood sugar levels, and metabolism are all regulated by the endocrine system. Consuming alcohol in excess interrupts the communicative processes between the endocrine, nervous, and immune systems. This can cause hormonal complications that can develop into severe physiological and behavioral issues such as thyroid malfunctions, body growth defect, reproductive complications, a compromised immune system, bone disease, and cancers.

Emotions

People often consume alcohol to cope with emotions such as stress, overwhelm, anxiety, and depression. Alcohol can improve your mood in small to moderate quantities; however, in increased amounts, alcohol can cause your mood to worsen. Certain people may feel anxiety or depression after consuming only one alcoholic beverage, whereas others may not feel any depression from drinking a moderate amount. Because alcohol is a depressant, it is not uncommon to feel depressed after drinking. Although dopamine may reinforce your craving for alcohol, it can also interfere with the neurotransmitters that control our moods, like norepinephrine and serotonin. Over the long term, these brain changes can cause or worsen mental health issues like anxiety and depression.

Initial Detox

If you drink heavily on a regular basis, you may find that you experience serious withdrawal symptoms when you stop drinking. The length of time needed to detox from alcohol depends on how much you were drinking and whether you have detoxed from alcohol before. Four to five days is the average time that people tend to stop experiencing withdrawal once they stop consuming alcohol. Some common symptoms that you may experience while detoxing are sweating, tremors, anxiety, depression, irritability, increased heart rate, and nausea. In more severe cases that manifest as delirium tremens (DT), you may experience delusions, paranoia, hallucinations, increased body temperature, and even seizures.

TRACK YOUR CRAVINGS

Tracking your cravings can help you gain awareness of the situations, thoughts, and emotions that trigger you to drink. Use the following chart to document your cravings for at least a week in order to become aware of what is making you want to drink.

DATE	SITUATION	EMOTION	THOUGHTS
	What happened that made you feel upset/triggered/ disturbed/excited and made you want to drink?	How strong is your emotion on a scale from 1 to 10, where 1 is the least strong and 10 is the strongest?	What thoughts crossed your mind immediately after this situation occurred?

REWRITING YOUR ROUTINE AND CREATING RITUALS

For many of us, the habit of drinking has become so built in to our daily lives that quitting or reducing our alcohol intake can be quite challenging or even seem impossible. In an effort to break these habits, many people have found that rewriting their routines and creating new rituals has been helpful for them in their sobriety journey. Oftentimes, relapse occurs because the old ritual of drinking is so ingrained in our heads that it's hard to imagine anything different. For instance, we may be accustomed to having a drink when we get home from work, drinking when we go out to meet friends or dates, or drinking at family gatherings or when we are stressed.

What could you choose to do instead of drinking in these moments? Perhaps something that might provide some similar type of relief or comfort? For instance, when you get home from work, instead of drinking, you may choose to practice yoga, meditation, or breathing techniques. Alternatively, you may want to journal or reach out to a friend that is in recovery. Instead of meeting friends or dates at a bar, you may choose to meet them at a coffee shop, restaurant, or juice bar, or invite them to go for a walk. Instead of drinking at family gatherings, you may choose to inform your family members that you are quitting or cutting down on drinking and arrive prepared with your favorite nonalcoholic beverage. You may also choose to ask your family members if they would be okay with not having alcohol at the family gathering this year and choose some other activities to engage in together such as playing board games, going for a hike, or enjoying the outdoor garden or pets.

The following is a table that can help you see what your old drinking rituals/routines were. This will help you write over them in a way that promotes growth, stability, and your recovery.

TIMES/EVENTS WHEN I USED TO DRINK	HEALTHY ACTIVITY I WILL ENGAGE IN INSTEAD

TRACK YOUR EMOTIONS

The following is an exercise that will help you track your emotions around alcohol, sobriety, and recovery. Check in with yourself throughout the week whenever you notice yourself having a strong emotion and explore it in this table.

WHAT I'M FEELING	WHAT I USED TO DO WHEN I FELT THIS WAY	WHAT I DO NOW

In the Moment

You may notice that you feel overwhelmed while you work through this book and respond to the prompts. Feeling overwhelmed when being exposed to new ideas and gaining new awareness of the self is totally normal. In these moments, take time to check in with yourself. Find a comfortable seated position. Close your eyes and take 10 slow, deep breaths, focusing on the way the breath feels as it enters the nostrils, goes into the chest and belly, and then exits the belly, chest, and nostrils. If a thought enters your mind, or if you feel a strong emotion, you don't need to push it away. Just acknowledge it, gently let it go, and return your focus to your breath.

DEBRIEF AND DIGEST

In this chapter, we covered five key lessons:
- The brain plays a role in how thoughts and impulses can lead to excessive drinking.
- Serotonin and dopamine are neurotransmitters that reinforce alcohol dependence.
- Certain brain regions are responsible for memory, pleasure, and reward during alcohol cravings.
- Excess alcohol consumption adversely affects the body's hormones, emotions, and response to the initial detox process.
- Creating new rituals, rewriting your routines, and exploring mindfulness can help curb cravings.

SELF CHECK-IN

Take a deep breath, close your eyes, and explore how you are feeling after reading this chapter. What came up for you as you were reading? What emotions are you feeling right now?

Now take a moment to reflect on what you have read. What have you learned from this chapter? Have you gained any new insights or self-awareness? How do you think this new knowledge could be helpful for your sobriety journey going forward?

I can learn about myself.
I can be compassionate
with myself in the process.
Gaining awareness of my
triggers and core issues will
help me meet my goals.

Chapter 4

KNOW WHY YOU'RE DRINKING

Cultivating self-awareness is an essential part of a successful recovery. In this chapter, you will learn to identify your triggers—or, in other words, you will come to understand what makes you want to drink. You will also start to identify what your core issues are, which are often rooted in challenging experiences you had earlier in life. And lastly, you will set your own goals for treatment, such as how long you would like to maintain sobriety.

DRINKING TRIGGERS

In order to create a successful treatment plan, it is necessary to come to an understanding of what triggers you to drink. Triggers can be emotional, environmental, or both. Many people use alcohol to cope with these triggers because they have not learned more sustainable coping skills. This workbook will provide you with the tools and strategies to address and cope with your triggers when they arise.

Emotional Triggers: Emotional Drinking and Escape

- **Stress and anxiety:** People often drink in order to escape stress and anxiety. For example, drinking after a stressful workday is quite common and socially accepted, which is evident due to the prevalence of the "happy hour." Self-medicating anxiety with alcohol is also not uncommon, as alcohol tends to have a relaxing effect.
- **Boredom:** Many people also drink due to boredom. They may feel that they have nothing better to do, or they may be unhappy with their life or feel lonely. I have had clients who have shared that boredom has led them to relapse in the past. For many people, keeping busy helps them stay sober.
- **Trauma:** Some people may drink in order to cope with difficult memories or emotional states such as anxiety and depression that developed as a result of what happened in the past. They may have experienced what mental health professionals call a "big T trauma," such as war or physical, sexual, or emotional abuse, or a "little t trauma," such as being harassed or bullied at school or experiencing a breakup. Research shows that most alcoholics have had traumatic experiences in the past.
- **Childhood habits:** Addictive tendencies often start in childhood, perhaps as a response to traumatic experiences. Many alcoholics engaged in addictive behaviors prior to their first drink that may have involved food, relationships, emotional attachments, and sex. Having learned early on to self-medicate their emotions, these compulsive behaviors likely served as a stepping stone for substance use disorders later on in life.
- **Social drinking:** Many people feel uncomfortable when they attempt to abstain from alcohol at social gatherings because of the pressure to fit in or a fear of being different or standing out, and in order to please others. It's a normal human

instinct to want to fit in and belong to a group. However, this natural drive to fit in and belong can often make it challenging to maintain sobriety.

Environmental Triggers: Things in Your Environment That Make You Want to Drink

- **Parties and other social gatherings:** Alcohol tends to be widely available and consumed at most parties and other social gatherings in our culture, and people often start drinking in high school or as early as middle school. Many special occasions like weddings and most holidays involve some sort of tradition of drinking as well. The prevalence of social events that involve drinking may cause us to feel pressured to drink and make it likely that we will feel left out when we attempt to stay sober.

- **Social events at bars:** Bars can be a major trigger for many individuals who are attempting to abstain from alcohol. For many, socializing is centered around bars, and meeting people at the local pub or cocktail lounge is the primary way to connect with our friends. It's the place for after work beers, girls' nights out, and dates. For those who want to maintain sobriety, moving the center of their social life away from bars may feel challenging, and oftentimes they find that avoiding bars altogether, especially when they are early in their recovery, is necessary.

- **Empty cups and portion control:** For those who have a problem with alcohol, portion control can be quite challenging. You may have friends who have just one or two drinks, or who leave their drinks unfinished when they feel "done," but that tends to feel impossible to alcoholics. You may find that you intended to have only a drink or two, but you are unable to follow through with that intention once you have a couple drinks in you. You also may find it difficult to stop midway through a beverage, even if you know you have had enough. For many of us, once we get even a little bit of alcohol in our bodies, the craving response goes full force and takes control.

REFLECTION ON ALCOHOL-RELATED TRIGGERS

Figuring out what makes you want to drink plays an essential role in your goal of reducing alcohol usage. Gaining awareness of the cause of your cravings will strengthen your ability to abstain from drinking when you want to.

Think of a few times this week when you craved a drink. What happened before you got the craving? What emotions were you feeling? Where were you feeling these emotions in your body? What would drinking do for you in those scenarios? (For example, would drinking calm you down? Relieve stress or anxiety? Make you feel more comfortable in a social setting?)

_____

_____

_____

_____

_____

_____

_____

Now identify a few activities that could help solve the problem that drinking has thus far been solving for you. What other activities make you feel similarly to the way that drinking alcohol does? (For example, meditation, yoga, or another form of exercise that could help you relax and reduce stress or anxiety; or reaching out to a friend to help you feel supported and connected.)

_____

_____

_____

_____

_____

_____

WHAT'S GOING ON?

In addition to identifying your triggers, determining what your core issues are can also help you gain the self-awareness that you need in order to maintain sobriety. Core issues are limiting beliefs, unresolved trauma, unhealthy relationships, and mental health conditions that may be at the root of your addiction to alcohol. Once you identify your core issues, you will be able to better understand the source of your urge to drink and how best to manage it.

Some examples of how core issues may manifest are low self-esteem, unhealed trauma, codependency, anger, and difficulty with communication and setting boundaries. For example, experiencing some sort of trauma as a child, such as divorce or abuse, can cause one to have low self-esteem. These feelings of low self-worth make it difficult for them to feel comfortable interacting with other people when they are sober, so they drink in order to ease the discomfort.

EXPLORING YOUR CORE ISSUES

People often describe alcohol dependency as feeling like they have a big hole inside them that they use alcohol to fill up. The problem is that alcohol, while providing temporary relief, tends to just make the hole bigger over time. It may be helpful to understand our core issues as the aspects of our lives that have created this hole inside us. Understanding what created this hole is an important part of your journey toward getting sober.

Take a moment to reflect on what your core issues may be that lead you to drink. It may be helpful to visualize this hole that you fill up with alcohol—what are the issues hiding there in the shadows demanding to be fed? What do you think your main issues are that lead you to drink? Do you identify with any of the core issues mentioned earlier?

_____

_____

_____

_____

_____

In the Moment

It is common to feel overwhelmed after an alcoholic episode. Maybe you are experiencing shame or regret, or you are struggling with anxiety or feelings of sadness. In these moments, it can be very helpful to do things that activate your physical senses in order to center yourself in your body. Exposure to warm and cool temperatures can help reduce feelings of overwhelm. This is a skill that is often used to tolerate distress in dialectical behavioral therapy (DBT). Take some time out to take a hot bath or a cold shower. Notice how you feel before, during, and afterward. Offer yourself some forgiveness and compassion by using affirmations, meditation, or prayer. Talk with a friend or watch a funny movie if you are still feeling overwhelmed. Remind yourself that recovery is a process and you can always start again.

SET YOUR GOALS

I have found that setting goals has been supportive of my own recovery as well as my clients' recovery. Short- and long-term goals can assist in providing motivation as well as a template of what we would like our futures to look like.

Many individuals who want to cut down on their alcohol use may not be fully aware of what their short-term goals are until their therapist, sponsor, or mentor provides them with the opportunity to identify them. When working with individuals who desire to cut down on or quit using alcohol, inquiring about and gaining awareness of short-term goals can be a stepping stone to reaching their long-term goals.

Short-term goals, such as aiming to reduce weekly or daily alcohol consumption or entirely abstaining from alcohol for a certain period of time, have helped many of my clients uncover what their longer-term goals are. Long-term goals can start to seem more achievable when clients are able to identify and attain short-term goals. Having goals in mind can also help us refrain from "autopilot" behavior and succumbing to triggers, because it encourages mindfulness of our intentions and behaviors.

The following exercise will help you identify some of your short-term and long-term goals.

SET SHORT- AND LONG-TERM GOALS

Take a moment to reflect on some of your short-term goals. Do you want to quit drinking indefinitely, or would you prefer to quit temporarily or cut down on your alcohol consumption? Do you want to try going to some recovery meetings offered by groups such as Alcoholics Anonymous (AA), Recovery Dharma, or SMART Recovery? Do you want to try incorporating daily exercise or mindfulness practices? Write down your short-term goals.

Now take a moment to reflect on some of your long-term goals. What would you like your relationship with alcohol to be like in the future? Do you want to work through a recovery program or become a sponsor or mentor in a program yourself? Do you have any long-term self-care goals such as exercise, nutrition, or mindfulness goals? What would help you in maintaining your sobriety? Write down your long-term goals.

DEBRIEF AND DIGEST

In this chapter, we covered five key lessons:
- Cultivating self-awareness is an essential part of a successful recovery.
- Uncomfortable emotions, stress and anxiety, boredom, childhood habits, trauma, and social drinking are a few of the things that lead us to drink.
- Parties, social events at bars, and empty cups can all be environmental triggers.
- Identifying your triggers and core issues can help you gain the self-awareness that you need in order to maintain sobriety.
- Setting short- and long-term goals helps prevent "autopilot" behavior and succumbing to triggers.

SELF CHECK-IN

What have you learned from reading this chapter? Do you have a greater understanding of your own personal triggers and core issues? How might this new knowledge be helpful for your sobriety and recovery?

How are you feeling about what you have learned? Take a breath, close your eyes, and scan your body. What emotions are you feeling right now? Where do you feel them in your body? Try to breathe into those places and send them kind and compassionate thoughts.

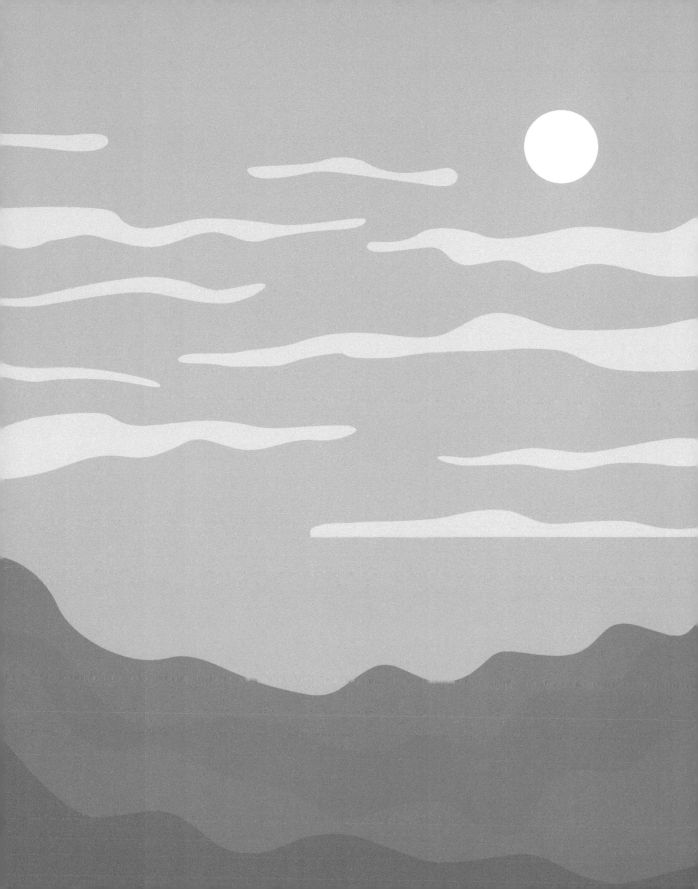

PART 2

COPING SKILLS AND RECOVERY

I can learn new skills. I am open
to learning. I can recover.
The new skills that I learn
will support me in my recovery.

I am open and willing
to learn and implement
new skills and tools that
will help me manage my
emotions, improve my
relationships, and maintain
my sobriety.

Chapter 5

YOUR JOURNEY TOWARD SOBRIETY

In this chapter, we will discuss the many different ways in which you can treat and manage alcoholism and how you can use these tools to help you live a better life. We will learn about therapeutic approaches and recovery programs such as cognitive behavioral therapy (CBT), mindfulness/meditation, distress tolerance, interpersonal therapy, and AA. We will also learn about medication-based approaches such as antianxiety and antidepressant medications.

COGNITIVE BEHAVIORAL THERAPY

CBT is a structured, evidence-based approach used by many mental health professionals that focuses on identifying, examining, and making the connection between triggering situations, emotions, thoughts, physical sensations, and core beliefs. It is one of the most popular psychotherapy approaches to treating alcoholism and addiction and has also been shown to be effective in treating depression, anxiety, anger, stress, and more.

The key idea in CBT is that our thoughts, feelings, and behaviors are all connected. For instance, if a person has negative thoughts about themselves, it may lead to feelings of shame and loneliness, which may then lead to behavior like excessive drinking to numb the pain. The goal of CBT is to identify the patterns in our thoughts, feelings, and behaviors and find healthy solutions to our problems. CBT differs from other forms of talk therapy in that it is specifically focused on solving problems in the here and now rather than focusing on the past and underlying reasons why you may be having these problems. CBT is often a great therapeutic tool in addition to other forms of talk therapy and recovery support. It can be used in group and individual therapy, and there are also workbooks that you can purchase and work through on your own.

Why CBT?

CBT is a structured form of therapy that helps people become more aware of their emotions (such as anger, sadness, anxiety, frustration, and shame). CBT can provide us with the tools to change our emotional state by changing the way that we think. For example, situations like bad traffic or a conversation with a boss or coworker that may trigger feelings of anger or stress can be looked at in a rational manner that can help us have more control over our emotions.

One of the main concepts of CBT is core beliefs, also known as limiting beliefs that we have about ourselves, others, and the world. These limiting beliefs are often unconscious and tend to be formed in childhood, though they often frame the way that we see things. Some examples of core beliefs about ourselves are "I am shameful," "I am not worthy," and "I am a failure."

Another concept is "automatic thoughts"—the thoughts that we have right away when a situation occurs. Automatic thoughts are often cognitive distortions, or nonrational thoughts, that result in an unwanted or unpleasant emotion.

One frequently used CBT tool is learning to identify cognitive distortions, such as all-or-nothing thinking, and learning to reframe these unhelpful thoughts. We will get into cognitive distortions later in the book.

CBT is time-based, which is helpful for those who don't want to feel like they're forever tied to therapy. It is focused on addressing specific problems in the present, so once you have learned the tools you need to work with that particular issue, you are free to move on.

How Does It Work?

CBT can help you manage drinking triggers and underlying issues by helping you identify—and change—the thought patterns that lead to your drinking. Central to this approach is addressing our limiting or core beliefs, which often act as unconscious triggers that make us want to drink. In CBT, we can identify and challenge limiting beliefs by using what is called "the downward spiral technique." The idea is to look at a limiting belief in a rational manner, trying to find evidence to support whether it is—or is not—true, and exploring other possibilities for the truth. In using logic to disprove a limiting belief, the feelings that lead a person to drink lose some of their fuel.

Another frequently used tool in CBT includes "the thought record," which helps individuals identify situations that trigger them to feel unpleasant emotions, the "automatic thoughts" associated with those emotions, and how to reframe those thoughts to produce a more balanced emotional outcome. CBT also works with cognitive distortions by helping people identify and interrupt negative thought patterns such as mind reading, negative filtering, overgeneralization, and jumping to conclusions. Identifying these cognitive distortions can reduce the power that our thoughts tend to hold over us. By working to find concrete solutions to problems addressing what is often the source of our behavior—our thoughts—CBT is a powerful tool to break the cycle of problem drinking.

CBT CHECK-IN

Sometimes learning about new skills can uncover buried feelings and beliefs and make us feel anxious or afraid. Take a moment to reflect on the previous section. How do you feel about using CBT to manage your triggers and cravings for alcohol? How do you feel when you think about exploring your limiting or core beliefs, automatic thoughts, and cognitive distortions? Are you open and willing to try these new skills? Is there anything preventing you from wanting to try them?

_____

_____

_____

_____

_____

_____

_____

_____

OTHER TYPES OF TREATMENT

Although CBT is considered by many to be the most effective medication-free method to help treat alcoholism, there are other techniques and tools out there such as DBT, mindfulness/meditation, distress tolerance, interpersonal therapy (IPT), and AA and other recovery programs.

Mindfulness/Meditation

Mindfulness can be defined as simply being present in the current moment, which may sound simple, but many people find it incredibly challenging. It can be cultivated through simple practices like checking in with ourselves throughout the day and taking a few deep breaths, or through more formal practices like meditation. In meditation, one concentrates on the breath, the body, a visualization, or a mantra in order to focus attention and calm the reactive "monkey mind." Just 5 to 10 minutes of meditation holds the potential to transform an uncomfortable emotional state. According to research, yoga has also been shown to improve well-being and reduce depression and anxiety.

Distress Tolerance

Examples of incidents that may cause a person to feel distress can range from something as seemingly benign as traffic on the highway or a difficult workday to a traumatic life event such as an assault or a loved one dying. People who have a difficult time tolerating distress have been found to be more likely to have drinking problems. Studies have found that learning to tolerate distress is likely to play a significant role in one's ability to abstain from alcohol.

Distress tolerance is one of the key components of DBT. If you are interested in learning a variety of distress tolerance skills, you may want to find a psychotherapist or group therapist who specializes in DBT.

Interpersonal Therapy

IPT is a highly structured and time-limited approach (typically 12 to 16 weeks) that focuses on relationships, attachment issues, and solving interpersonal problems in order to provide symptom relief. Although it has many similarities to CBT, it focuses more on feelings and relationships than thoughts. Researchers have suggested that IPT is most effective for recovery when it emphasizes the significance of developing meaningful roles in society, developing relationships with people who are sober, utilizing relational aspects of motivational interviewing, and cultivating self-soothing capabilities through the therapeutic relationship.

Alcoholics Anonymous

AA is a well-known 12-step recovery program founded in 1935 that focuses on developing a relationship with a higher power, a sponsor, and the community of AA. There are a wide variety of AA meetings in many areas such as speaker meetings, book study meetings, meditation meetings, and affinity meetings based on gender, for people who identify as LGBTQ+, or for atheists/agnostics. Research evaluating the effectiveness of AA has been varied; however, some variables such as level of attendance and effort have been shown to be predictive of the programs' outcome. Many of my clients, peers, and I have used 12-step programs to support us in our recovery.

Other Recovery Programs

Some people find that they do not quite fit in with AA, feel alienated by its emphasis on a higher power, or, depending on where they live, cannot find meetings in which they feel welcome. Luckily, there are many other recovery programs and communities that have developed over the last several years, offering an alternative to AA that some may find to be more in line with their beliefs and identities. For example, SMART Recovery (short for Self-Management and Recovery Training) is a secular and research-based program based on CBT. Recovery Dharma is a Buddhist-based recovery program that is open to people struggling with addictive behaviors of all kinds. Other alternative programs include Women in Recovery and LifeRing Secular Recovery, among others.

MEDICATIONS

Many people who have problems with drinking also struggle with mental health issues like depression and anxiety, and some may benefit from psychiatric medication. Like any medical treatment, there are pros and cons to utilizing medications to manage your emotions and sobriety. Medication may help you move away from alcohol use more quickly and help you feel less depressed or anxious, but it may have unpleasant short- and long-term side effects. It may be difficult to reduce your dependency on or stop taking the medication, depending on how much and how long you have taken it. When deciding whether medication is right for you, it's important to always have a medical doctor or psychiatrist evaluate you.

Antidepressants

People who are diagnosed with major depressive disorder (MDD) are more likely to develop a dependence on alcohol, and those who are dependent on alcohol are more likely to develop MDD. Selective serotonin reuptake inhibitors (SSRIs) are the most commonly prescribed antidepressants to treat MDD. Some SSRIs to treat depression have been shown to be helpful in clinical trials in calming one of the triggers that may lead to drinking episodes. However, many studies have shown inconsistent outcomes for the use of SSRIs in treating AUD; some studies show that SSRIs can actually increase alcohol dependence. Different people can have very different responses to the same medications, so it is always important to closely monitor your symptoms with the help of a professional.

Antianxiety Medication

Anxiety disorders are more common among women than men. Antianxiety medication may help reduce anxiety, thereby lessening triggers that could lead to drinking. For individuals who have a comorbid diagnosis of PTSD, anxiety, and AUD, SSRIs have been proven to be effective, although they should be monitored closely because SSRIs can cause individuals to drink more.

Although treating AUD with antianxiety medications has been effective for some, the evidence to support the use of antianxiety medication to treat alcohol dependence alone is weak. A couple of recent studies showed improvement in symptoms, but many other studies did not show any improvement. In addition, many people reported experiencing negative sexual side effects from the medication. It is also possible that the studies with successful outcomes were skewed due to being funded by pharmaceutical companies.

In the Moment

The following is an exercise you can use to manage any overwhelming feelings that may occur in the moment or shortly after an alcoholic episode.

Take some time for yourself, finding a comfortable seated position. Close your eyes and connect with your breath and your body. Notice what is going on with your breath. Is it long or short? Choppy or smooth? Now notice what is happening with your body. Where do you feel emotions in your body? Breathe through them. Place your hands on your heart and send yourself some loving thoughts, compassion, and forgiveness. Tell yourself some words of encouragement for moving forward and getting through this. Remind yourself that feelings are temporary. See what it feels like to try to relate to yourself as if you are a beloved friend or family member. Send yourself love as you would to someone you care deeply about. This could be as simple as silently telling yourself "I love you."

DEBRIEF AND DIGEST

In this chapter, we covered five key lessons:

- You can cope with and treat alcohol dependence through recovery programs and/or using therapeutic and medication-based approaches.
- Therapeutic tools like CBT, mindfulness, distress tolerance, and IPT can improve your life and support your sobriety.
- There are many different community-based recovery programs available, including AA (with affinity meetings based on gender, for people who identify as LGBTQ+, or for atheists/agnostics), SMART Recovery, and Recovery Dharma.
- There are pros and cons to medication-based recovery approaches.
- You can manage overwhelming feelings in the midst of or after an alcoholic episode by grounding yourself and practicing self-compassion.

SELF CHECK-IN

Take a moment to reflect on the emotions you are feeling. Where are you feeling them in your body? It's not uncommon to feel some apprehension or fear when learning about new treatments that are likely to promote change. Close your eyes and sit with whatever you are feeling right now. Breathe.

Take a moment to reflect on what you have read in this chapter. Did you learn anything new? Are there any particular approaches that sound appealing to you?

_____

_____

_____

_____

_____

_____

_____

_____

_____

_____

_____

_____

_____

_____

_____

_____

_____

_____

_____

_____

_____

_____

_____

_____

_____

_____

_____

_____

_____

_____

_____

_____

_____

_____

I am not my emotions.
I can observe my emotions.
Observing my emotions
will empower me to have
more control over my
responses to my emotions
and support me
in my recovery.

Chapter 6

CHALLENGE YOUR THOUGHTS

Feeling overwhelmed by emotions can lead to drinking as a means of escape. Learning to separate yourself from your emotions by observing your thoughts when they come up can reduce their intensity. Once you observe your emotions, you can try to sit with them instead of running from them, which lessens the power that they hold over you and builds your resiliency. This chapter will offer tools to help you do just that.

BREAKING THE NEGATIVE THINKING CIRCLE

Those who struggle with alcoholism often have negative thought patterns that can dominate how they think about themselves, their lives, and their relationship with alcohol. These negative thought patterns can cause a great deal of unnecessary mental anguish, which can potentially contribute to why an individual may desire to drink in excess. In CBT, we identify cognitive distortions, or dysfunctional ways of thinking that tend to result in unbalanced emotions. Some examples of cognitive distortions are black-and-white thinking, overgeneralizing, and jumping to conclusions. Many of our negative thought patterns can fit into more than one category of cognitive distortion. For instance, a certain thought may fit into the category of black-and-white thinking as well as jumping to conclusions. Identifying our thoughts as cognitive distortions will help us gain the awareness that will take the power away from those thoughts. Reframing these thoughts with a more rational lens will alleviate a lot of the emotional charge associated with the original thought.

Black-and-White Thinking

Black-and-white thinking, also known as all-or-nothing thinking, is when we tend to think in ways that are either all one way or all another way, and we are unable or unwilling to see any grey area or middle ground. In other words, when people engage in black-and-white thinking, their thoughts are full of absolutes, such as "I'm either perfect, or I'm a failure." If you are thinking in terms of "always," "never," "impossible," "perfect," or "ruined," you may be engaging in black-and-white thinking. Some examples of black-and-white thinking are being insulted by someone and believing that you are not worthy of respect, pushing people away or ending relationships because people aren't "perfect" all the time, or accidentally doing something wrong at your job and concluding that you are unemployable and a bad person. Black-and-white thinking can result in us activating limiting beliefs like "I'm not good enough," "I am shameful," or "I'm unlovable." Taking our limiting beliefs to heart can result in overwhelming emotions of sadness, anger, and anxiety. When we feel flooded with emotions like these, alcoholic episodes are much more likely to occur.

Anecdote

Crystal is in college and got a poor grade on her biology test. Because of the poor grade, Crystal concluded she is not intelligent and is a failure in life.

Explanation

Crystal is unable to see that just because she scored poorly on a test does not mean that she is not smart and can't do well on another test or in other areas of academic achievement. People experiencing black-and-white thinking may be unable to see what their strengths are and see poor test results only as a general failure in life. For instance, Crystal may be skilled at researching and writing but not so skilled at test taking. Or perhaps the subject matter of this particular test was more challenging than other tests. Either way, this type of thinking can lead to entertaining limiting beliefs such as "I'm a failure," which can cause her to feel sad or angry and potentially lead to an alcoholic episode. Learning to see the grey area can help Crystal feel more balanced emotionally and reduce any potential triggers that may result in drinking.

Exercise

Can you think of any times when you have experienced black-and-white thinking? What happened? How did you feel? What were your thoughts associated with your feelings and the event? How can you reframe your thoughts in order to have a more balanced outcome?

EVENT	What happened that caused you to experience black-and-white thinking?			
EMOTIONS	What emotions did you feel? How strong where your emotions on a scale from 1 to 100 (where 1 is the least strong and 100 is the strongest)?			
THOUGHTS	What was your black-and-white thought? For example, "I failed the driving test, and I will never be able to drive."			
THOUGHT REFRAME	What would be a more balanced way to think about it? What is the grey area or middle ground?			
EMOTIONS	What emotions are you feeling now after reframing your thought?			

Overgeneralizing

Overgeneralizing, or the tendency to assume broad truths based on limited information, is another example of a cognitive distortion that is addressed in CBT. Overgeneralization, like other cognitive distortions, can lead us to negative emotional states that can potentially trigger us to drink. Like black-and-white thinking, people who tend to overgeneralize are likely to use words like "always," "never," "nobody," and "everybody," even when they are not necessarily true. We may predict the outcome of something based on just one instance of it. For instance, we had one bad date, so we conclude we will never find love. Or we had one bad job interview and are convinced that we'll never find a job and our career is going nowhere. Sometimes people overgeneralize because they are consciously exaggerating for dramatic effect, but for many of us, it reflects how we see the world and we actually believe these thoughts. This line of thinking can intensify emotions like anger, frustration, or sadness and can potentially lead us to drink in order to soothe our emotions.

Anecdote

Samira feels like her partner, Jess, occasionally tunes her out or talks over her when they get into a disagreement. Feeling unheard or invalidated, she tells her significant other that they *never* listen when she is talking to them.

Explanation

Telling Jess that they never listen is likely to put them on the defensive, which could lead to intensification of the disagreement. Samira may be exaggerating her partner's behavior for dramatic effect; however, this statement probably makes Samira seem unfair and irrational to Jess, causing more of a rift between them. The fighting that may ensue could lead to even more intensified emotions and an alcoholic episode, furthering the cycle of negative thought patterns, overwhelming emotions, and drinking.

If Samira felt that she was not being listened to and instead said something like "I feel like you are not hearing me" or "Oftentimes I feel that you are not listening to me," is it likely that their disagreement and the outcome of it would be less intense?

In order for Samira to prevent herself from overgeneralizing, it would be helpful for her to check how accurate her statement was. Does it really "always" or "never" happen? Or would it be more accurate to say that it "sometimes" or "often" happens?

Exercise

Think of a recent time when you overgeneralized—perhaps when you used the word "always" or "never." Was it really the case that this situation "always" or "never" occurred? Or would it be more accurate to say that it happened often or rarely? What is a more accurate statement about the situation? How could making this new statement potentially change the way you feel about the situation?

_____

_____

_____

_____

_____

_____

_____

Jumping to Conclusions

Another negative thought pattern, or cognitive distortion, that has the potential to trigger people to drink in excess is jumping to conclusions. Like it sounds, this is when an individual makes assumptions about something or someone without having all the information necessary. Another way to think of jumping to conclusions is taking an insubstantial amount of evidence and blowing it up in your mind as though it provides a substantial amount of evidence. Some examples of jumping to conclusions are assuming that your date is an irresponsible jerk because he was a few minutes late, assuming a parent has died when you have not heard back from them, or assuming people are saying negative things about you when you walk into a room. Jumping to conclusions can unnecessarily lead us into unpleasant emotional states like anger and sadness, which can cause us to drink if we do not properly address them.

Anecdote

Cassie's significant other has not answered the phone for a few hours. Because their partner is not answering the phone, Cassie convinces themself that their partner is having an affair or they are angry with Cassie.

Explanation

Concluding that their partner is cheating on Cassie when they don't answer the phone could lead Cassie to become suspicious, mistrustful, and angry. These feelings, if not taken care of in a healthy way, may lead to drinking in order to cope with them. Cassie could also end up accusing their partner of cheating without any substantial evidence, which would likely result in even more heightened emotions and potentially cause a rift in the relationship. The heightened emotions from fighting could also trigger Cassie to drink even more.

What can help prevent Cassie from jumping to conclusions? If they notice that they are feeling upset, Cassie can take a moment to consider the situation that caused the feeling, thoughts, and beliefs that Cassie automatically connected to that situation. They can try to consider all of the options for what could have happened before they decided on one option for sure. Cassie can also question or examine any thought or belief that sounds off or like it may be extreme.

Exercise

The exercise that follows will help you gain a better understanding of what jumping to conclusions is. Read the examples of jumping to conclusions in the following chart and then come up with some of your own explanations for what could have happened or what will happen.

EXAMPLE OF JUMPING TO CONCLUSIONS	OTHER EXPLANATIONS FOR WHAT COULD HAVE HAPPENED OR WHAT COULD HAPPEN
Because my partner did not answer the phone, they are cheating on me.	*My partner may have fallen asleep, their phone may have died, or they may be on the other line with someone.*
Because I haven't been to the dentist in years, they are going to tell me all my teeth are rotten and they all need to be pulled.	
Because I have been drinking a lot in the past year, that means I am a bad person.	
If I have to ask for help, that means I am weak.	
My boss looked at me strangely, so that means she is going to fire me.	

CONFRONT YOUR THOUGHTS

Through CBT, you can learn how to challenge your thoughts and change the way you think about your relationship with yourself and your emotions, which can have a profound effect on your relationship with alcohol. Rather than fighting with your thoughts, arguing with them, believing them, or trying to detach yourself from them, you will be able to gain understanding and accept that they are just thoughts.

Oftentimes we believe our thoughts without realizing it, even if they are not rational. For instance, your initial thought when someone is driving too slowly in front of you may be that the driver must be rude or incompetent. If you take a moment to examine and challenge your thought, you may consider that this driver may be new in town, they may be lost, or they may be feeling unwell. Considering other possibilities for why this person is driving slower than you think they should can help soften your emotional response.

Our thoughts may *feel* true, but that doesn't mean they *are* true. Taking time to become mindful of our thoughts can help us examine and challenge them, which will lessen their power over us and cultivate a more harmonious emotional state.

EXPLORE FOR EVIDENCE

A powerful tool for confronting our thoughts is exploring them for evidence. Identify a situation recently where a particular thought made you want to drink. What happened? What were your initial thoughts when that event occurred? Is there evidence to support your thought or belief? Is there evidence to support other thoughts or beliefs?

Journaling through Recovery

Often, people in recovery can find significant breakthroughs in journaling. While journaling may come easy for some, other people may find the idea of writing on a blank page daunting. Utilizing prompts to explore your thoughts and feelings can make your experience much easier and more fulfilling by providing direction for your exploration.

Some journal prompt ideas after an alcoholic episode:

* What happened? What are my thoughts about it? How am I feeling?

* Who can I reach out to for support? What kind of support do I need?

* What steps can I take today to be kind and gentle with myself?

* What happened before that may have triggered a setback?

* What are the emotions I am feeling right now?

* Am I blaming myself for this slipup and why?

* How am I going to take care of myself this week?

* What are some of my strengths and positive qualities?

It is helpful to remind yourself of your strengths after an alcoholic episode. Your support system—such as sober or supportive friends, members of recovery communities, or family members—is one of those strengths that can support you in your recovery. It's important to also remember that recovery is a journey, and an alcoholic episode is not the end of your recovery; you can always start again, move forward, and care for yourself. It's also pertinent to take note of what may have triggered you to drink this time so that you can take steps to care for yourself in a healthy way the next time you are triggered in a similar way. Self-awareness is key in supporting your sobriety and recovery, and journaling is a great tool in achieving this.

MY THOUGHTS ARE NOT ME

The following exercises are tools that can assist you in responding to your anxious thoughts in a healthy way and will support your recovery and sobriety.

Just a Thought: It's Just a Thought, Not a Fact

When you feel some type of emotional disturbance like anger, sadness, or anxiety, take some time to notice which thoughts are associated with those emotions. Remind yourself that they are just thoughts and not facts. How do you feel after telling yourself that?

Thought Power: Find a Way to Reduce the Power Your Thoughts Have Over You

Take a moment to observe your thoughts. What are you thinking? What stories are you internalizing about yourself or your situation? How is it making you feel? Where do you feel it in your body? Mindfully observing your thoughts like this is a powerful way to reduce the power they have over you.

Counteract a Thought: Find a Way to Challenge a Negative Thought

Bring to mind a negative thought you are having right now, or one that you have regularly. How is it making you feel? Is there any evidence to support that thought? Can you think of any other possibilities? Try coming up with a more rational or positive thought so that you feel more balanced emotionally.

Thought Evaluation: Is It Helpful, Truthful, or Important?

Take a moment to evaluate your thought. Ask yourself: Is it helpful, truthful, or important? If it is none of those things, are you willing to let the thought go?

Thought Detachment: Allow the Thought to Float Away

Find a comfortable seated position and sit up straight. Close your eyes. Bring your awareness to your breath, focusing on its quality. Is it long or short? Choppy or smooth? Deepen your breaths. If a thought comes up, notice it without judgment and allow it to float by like a cloud in the sky.

Worry Time: Set Aside Designated Time to Worry

When you notice that you are feeling worried or anxious, it can be helpful to visualize a box or container for that worry and put it aside for later. Schedule a time that would work for you to deal with your worries, and give yourself permission to wait until that time to think about them.

In the Moment

The following exercise will help you manage the overwhelming feelings that may occur in the moment, or shortly after or before an alcoholic episode.

When you notice overwhelming feelings coming up, reach out to a few different friends via phone. If you are unable to get in touch with anyone, go for a long walk until your feelings have lessened. Breathe as you walk and really feel the connection of your feet to the ground and the feeling of your body walking. Notice any plants or trees surrounding you. Notice the sky. Breathe. If you are able to get in contact with a friend or fellow member of a recovery program, you can also walk while you are speaking with them. Moving your body, being out in nature, and connecting with a trusted friend are all powerful ways to get out of our heads and manage our emotions.

DEBRIEF AND DIGEST

In this chapter, we covered five key lessons:
- Developing the ability to observe thoughts and making it a habit can assist you in maintaining your sobriety.
- You can learn to identify negative thought patterns, or cognitive distortions, that often lead to negative emotional states that may trigger us to drink.
- Some cognitive distortions include overgeneralizations, jumping to conclusions, and black-and-white thinking.
- Journaling can help you maintain your sobriety as you explore your motives for drinking and gain self-awareness.
- Reaching out to friends or going on a mindful walk when you are feeling overwhelmed will help reduce the power that your thoughts have over you.

SELF CHECK-IN

Take a moment to reflect on how you are feeling emotionally. Are there any differences from the emotions you experienced in the previous chapters? On a scale from 1 to 10 (where 1 is the least emotional charge and 10 is the most emotional charge), how strong does your emotion feel now?

Now take a moment to reflect on what you have read in this chapter. Did you learn anything new or different? What did you learn that you could apply to your sobriety and recovery? How might you apply these tools in different areas of your life?

_____

_____

_____

_____

_____

_____

_____

_____

_____

_____

_____

_____

_____

_____

_____

_____

_____

_____

_____

_____

I am not my emotions. I can observe my emotions. I can examine my emotions and change the thoughts that are connected to them to feel more empowered.

Chapter 7

HANDLING DIFFICULT EMOTIONS

Dealing with difficult emotions can be a challenge for many women. Sadness, fear, self-doubt, guilt, and anxiety are all normal feelings, but oftentimes we feel like they are dominating our lives. These strong, unpleasant emotions can lead to unhealthy coping mechanisms like drinking in an attempt to make them go away. When we learn to replace unhealthy ways of coping with healthy behaviors, we can gain more control over our emotions and thereby our behaviors.

WHEN YOU WANT TO RUN AWAY

Avoidance is a built-in tendency that is related to our brain's natural instinct to escape pain and bad experiences. It is totally normal, and everyone does it to some extent; the key is to not allow our avoidant tendencies to create negative consequences in our lives. Avoidant behavior may look like isolating yourself from people you love, shopping to excess, procrastination, binge-watching TV, sinking into a depression, or turning to alcohol to cope.

Some skills that can help us face our emotions instead of running from them are learning to accept our feelings, standing our ground in the face of difficult or uncomfortable feelings, and expressing our feelings. Coping tools and practices like mindfulness and CBT teach us how to "sit with" or be present with our feelings, observe them, and challenge the thoughts that are connected to them. In CBT, if we think negative thoughts, we will feel negative emotions, and then we will act in ways that may have negative consequences. In DBT there is a concept called "radical acceptance" that helps individuals accept their feelings and the situations they are in instead of running away from them. Acceptance is *not* approval of our unhappiness or getting to a point of being okay with or liking our difficulties. Instead, it is acknowledging the facts and recognizing that when we refuse to accept our present reality for what it is, we add to our suffering. This is a powerful tool that is supportive of recovery and can prompt us to accept "what is." We can also express our feelings by journaling, by using nonviolent communication techniques such as "I feel" statements, and by engaging in a creative activity such as art, music, or writing.

Once we have a collection of tools under our belts, we will feel much more supported in managing our emotions and will thereby find it easier to maintain our sobriety.

RECOGNIZE WHEN YOU RUN

The following exercise will help you recognize that running away from your emotions is only fueling your unhealthy coping strategies. Identify 2 to 3 situations that you drank over in the past, as well as the emotions that you were experiencing as a result of those situations.

SITUATIONS I DRANK OVER IN THE PAST	EMOTIONS I WAS RUNNING AWAY FROM

ACCEPT YOUR FEELINGS

Accepting your feelings can be of great help in managing your emotions and maintaining your sobriety. Learning to work with and through your emotions rather than constantly trying to fight them may seem counterintuitive, but by accepting that difficult emotions are inevitable in life, you can gain the ability to stay grounded during even the most turbulent times, rather than allowing your uncomfortable feelings to derail your progress toward long-term sobriety.

Accepting our emotions doesn't mean we are acquiescing to them or giving up. Rather, acceptance can help us create more harmony in our lives by reducing the resistance that we have to feeling our emotions. Resisting can oftentimes make things more painful than they need to be. As Carl Jung, the well-known Swedish psychologist, famously proclaimed, "What you resist persists." Making the choice to accept, observe, and sit with our emotions can lessen the power that they tend to hold over us when we avoid them, thereby increasing our ability to cope with triggers that may have previously led us to drink. If we are able to find the courage to feel our feelings rather than pushing them away, we are then able to respond to them with wisdom.

Inviting Difficult Emotions

The first step in accepting our emotions is learning to invite our difficult emotions to the so-called table rather than attempting to push them away. In inviting our challenging feelings, we can essentially "make friends" with them rather than thinking of them as our enemies. By allowing our uncomfortable emotions in, they will dissipate much quicker and feel more tolerable. So, the next time you notice a challenging feeling or multitude of challenging feelings coming up, try saying to it/them something like "welcome friend(s)!" or "hello, anxiety," or "I see you, sadness," and notice the difference in your emotional state.

Bring Compassion to Your Emotions

The next step in coming to truly accept our emotions is cultivating compassion for ourselves and our emotions. It can be helpful to affirm our own emotions by saying statements to ourselves and to our emotions that demonstrate empathy for them, such as "Feeling this way is really hard for you," or "I care about you." You can also add a mind-body component of compassion to your practice by putting your hands over your heart and connecting with your heart center, breathing and saying affirmative statements to yourself and to your emotions (e.g., "I know this hurts. . . . Feeling this way can be very uncomfortable.").

Validate Yourself

Sometimes we may feel a sense of shame about our feelings and are hard on ourselves because we think we "should" feel differently. Validating our own emotions can help us accept them and decrease the resistance we may feel toward them, again lessening their power over us. One way we can validate our own emotions is by saying to ourselves, "It makes sense that you feel this way. Anyone who had this happen to them would feel this way." We can also take up activities like journaling, drawing, or songwriting to validate and express our feelings.

Get Curious about Your Emotions

If we approach our emotions with curiosity rather than judgment, we will often learn important things about ourselves that can help us on our healing journey. A great way to do this is to literally "sit with" our emotions by sitting in a meditative posture, cross-legged on the floor or on a chair with both feet on the ground. Close your eyes and notice where you are feeling your emotions in your body. Become curious about what it feels like, what the temperature of the emotion would be if it were a temperature, what the texture of it would be if it were a texture, and what the color it would be if it were a color. Give that emotion some attention and breathe into that area of your body for 5 to 10 minutes. Then notice how that practice impacted your emotions and if you learned anything new.

HANDS ON HEART

When you feel a challenging emotion coming on, take some time and space to just notice it. Find a comfortable seated position, place your hands over your heart, and say affirmations to yourself silently or out loud. For example, "Hello, sadness. I'm letting you in," or "I know feeling this way is hard for you." Breathe and allow yourself to feel your feelings, sending them thoughts or words of love and compassion. You can also use visualization to surround your heart with a warm light, bathing it with love and understanding.

STAND YOUR GROUND

Feeling overwhelmed, having a desire to run away from emotions, avoiding feeling your feelings, and drinking to dull the senses can all pose serious challenges for those who are on the road to recovery. Using CBT tools can help you when you are feeling overwhelmed by your emotions and are tempted to run away from them, avoid them altogether, or turn to alcohol.

CBT is a widely used therapeutic approach that focuses on examining, observing, and challenging emotions, thoughts, and behaviors. A great deal of research has shown that using CBT can be just as effective as medication in treating many mental health conditions, including substance abuse, depression, anxiety, PTSD, and more. CBT tools like the thought record, awareness and examination of cognitive distortions, and exploring for exceptions have been shown to be helpful with managing the emotions that often lead us to drink. It takes courage to stand your ground with your emotions and to face them rather than running away. Adding these tools to your tool belt can give you the confidence and skills to do just that.

The following are some potential situations and emotions paired with strategies that will help you cope with difficult feelings in the moment.

Overwhelmed with Emotions

Being overwhelmed with emotions can be incredibly triggering for many people, especially people who have a history of alcohol dependence and are attempting to stop drinking. When we are overwhelmed, oftentimes there are one or more negative cognitions or thoughts associated with that feeling of overwhelm. Examining and challenging our thoughts that came about just before we began to feel overwhelmed can greatly reduce the emotional charge that we are feeling, thereby reducing our need to self-soothe with alcohol.

Strategy #1: Challenge Negative Thoughts

Think of a recent situation that caused you to feel overwhelmed. What happened? What were some of the thoughts that came to you right away when this event occurred? How would you characterize your thoughts? As we discussed in earlier chapters, cognitive distortions, or negative thought patterns, can often lead to feeling intense emotions. How could you challenge these negative thought patterns? Are there any other possibilities for what could have occurred?

Strategy #2: Use Your Breath

Another strategy for dealing with emotional overwhelm is breathing techniques. This technique would be more associated with mindfulness-based CBT rather than the classic version. Breathing exercises can calm down the sympathetic nervous system, or the fight-or-flight response, while helping us enter into our parasympathetic nervous system, which engages and allows for rest and relaxation.

FOCUS ON YOUR EXHALATION

Find a comfortable seated position. Begin to notice the quality of your breath. Now deepen your inhales and exhales. You may notice that as you observe your breath, it will naturally elongate. Now inhale to the count of 3 or 4 and exhale to the count of 3 or 4. After a few breaths, begin inhaling to the count of 3 or 4 and exhaling to the count of 6 or 8, so that you are exhaling twice as long as you inhale. Take 10 breaths, making the exhale twice as long as the inhale. Then go back to breathing equal amounts, inhaling to a count of 3 or 4 and exhaling to 3 or 4. Then, after a few breaths, when you are ready, slowly bring yourself back to the room and open your eyes, allowing the light to filter in.

Notice how you feel now. Do you feel any different from when you started?

Want to Run Away

Many of us have a desire to run from our emotions when they are unpleasant. How can we manage to stay present with our feelings even when they are challenging and even painful? Using mindfulness practices in this case can be extremely powerful. Mindfulness helps us sit and observe our emotions rather than run from them. By doing this, we may realize that perhaps our uncomfortable emotions aren't as bad as they seem. We can also recognize that our feelings are not necessarily good or bad—they just are. This realization may provide some relief while sitting with difficult emotions.

Strategy #1: Mindfulness

In order to be more present with our feelings, we can try sitting in meditation or doing mindful movement practices like yoga or tai chi. Other forms of exercise such as swimming, running, and dancing can also be very mindfulness-oriented, as long as you are paying attention to your senses and engaging your mind-body connection.

Strategy #2: Exceptions to the Rule

Perhaps you want to run away from your feelings because you are having rather harsh all-or-nothing thoughts. Take a moment to ask yourself, "Could it be possible that whatever I'm thinking is not true? Is there an exception to this thought? What is the best-case scenario in this situation?"

MINDFULLY CHECKING IN

Practicing mindfulness does not always require several minutes to sit quietly in formal meditation practice. A powerful form of mindfulness is simply taking time to check in with yourself throughout the day. You can set an hourly timer on your phone (I recommend using a gentle alarm or timer sound) to remind yourself to take a deep breath and ask yourself how you're feeling and what you might need. This is a great way to prevent "autopilot" behavior and to ensure you are making mindful, intentional decisions and actions.

How did that feel for you? Do you notice any difference in how you feel now versus before you did this exercise? How does your body feel after checking in?

Avoid Feelings

Avoiding unpleasant feelings can sometimes breed resentment, which can result in emotional outbursts. If we learn to go toward our feelings instead of avoiding them, it is likely we will find more of a sense of peace. Identifying our feelings is the first step toward facing them. Then, by using compassionate, nonviolent communication techniques (with others and ourselves), we can learn to express our feelings in an assertive, healthy manner, which will be more likely to get us the results we would like.

Strategy #1: Journaling

Journaling can be a very effective tool to help you face your feelings in a private manner before opening up to others about them. When you are journaling, you can contemplate your thoughts and feelings on your own, which can feel more comfortable to those who have a hard time expressing their feelings to others. Oftentimes journaling can help process and resolve the feelings.

Strategy #2: Share Your Feelings

We can share our feelings using compassionate, nonviolent communication strategies such as "I feel" statements. Many people may be afraid to share their feelings because they fear how other people will react. This fear and discomfort can drive us to drink. When we use "I feel" statements, the chances are higher that the person we are communicating with will react with less defensiveness and frustration, and we are more likely to feel heard, lessening the build-up of resentment.

"I FEEL" STATEMENTS

Take a moment to check in on how you feel. If you would like to, go ahead and write a few pages about it in your journal, or maybe even consider waiting 24 hours until you share your feelings to make sure it is necessary. After you have done those things, if you still feel that you would like to share your feelings, write down what you would like to say first. Instead of saying "You make me feel angry," say something like "I feel angry when you . . ." Notice the difference in how it feels for you and the person you are communicating with to share in that way. Now congratulate yourself mentally for sharing your feelings in an assertive manner.

Do you notice any difference in how you feel when you communicate this way? If you communicated to another person this way, how did they respond?

Drinking to Dull the Senses

Many of us drink to dull the senses and numb emotions. Numbing out is just another form of running away from discomfort. As mentioned before, exercising, talking it out with a friend or recovery buddy, confronting the emotion, having compassion for it, and meditating are all healthy strategies for finding relief from uncomfortable emotions.

Strategy #1: Thought Record

A thought record can reduce the emotional impact of a situation by helping us identify our triggers and question our initial thoughts and emotions associated with them. From there, we can investigate our "automatic thoughts" and see whether there is evidence to support them or any evidence against them. Then we can come up with a new thought or thoughts that lessen the emotional charge and may even produce a sense of empowerment. Afterward, we can rate our emotion compared to where it started and see how much it has changed as a result of altering our thoughts.

Strategy #2: Think It Through

If your recovery is wavering, make a list of the pros and cons of drinking. What would happen if you were to drink? What would happen if you avoided drinking for the time being? What are some other ways you can deal with your feelings? Once you think it through, you are likely to realize that the cons outweigh the pros and you will be able to brainstorm other options that will help with your feelings.

THOUGHT RECORD TO REDUCE INTENSITY OF EMOTIONS

Complete the following thought record in order to gain awareness of the thoughts that are connected to your emotions and reduce their intensity. You can make use of a chart like this whenever you would like to gain more control of your emotions.

After you complete it, reflect on what that process was like for you. Do you think it could be helpful to use going forward?

SITUATION	What event occurred that made you feel upset/triggered?	
EMOTION	What emotion(s) were you feeling and how intensely were you feeling them on a scale from 1 to 10?	
AUTOMATIC THOUGHTS	What were the first few thoughts that came into your mind when this situation occurred?	
EXAMINE THOUGHTS	Is there evidence for or against these thoughts?	
NEW THOUGHTS	What thought could you replace your automatic thought with that would make you feel more balanced?	
EMOTIONS	After replacing your automatic thought, how strongly do you feel the emotion you documented in row 2 on a scale from 1 to 10?	

Express Yourself

The habit of turning to alcohol during emotional turmoil can (and often does) develop from not properly expressing our feelings. Often, people will suppress their feelings because they don't want to feel them, are afraid to feel them, and fear sharing them with others.

Following are a few tips that will help you safely express your feelings. Expressing your feelings does not mean that you will get lost in them or that they will take over and get out of control. Feeling and expressing them is often the best way to let them out, which can lead to a sense of freedom to move on.

If you need to share your feelings with another person, using "I feel" statements can let others know how you feel and may also help you get your needs met. After you express your feelings, you can make a request if you would like to, such as "I would really appreciate it if you did not drink in my house." Learning to express your feelings and needs in a healthy manner will help you greatly with boundary setting, which many alcoholics, especially women, tend to struggle with.

Some other ways you can express your feelings are by journaling, making art or music, and calling up a trusted friend or recovery buddy and venting a bit about what has been going on. People struggling with anger often find it helpful to get aggression out by punching a pillow or punching bag.

In the Moment

The following is an exercise that you can use to manage/alleviate the overwhelming feelings that may occur in the moment or shortly after a binge drinking phase. Before you start, take a moment to notice your breath. Taking long, deep breaths can help reduce any anxiety or overwhelm that you may be feeling. When you feel that you have been able to connect with your breath, cultivate a sense of groundedness by making your way through these steps:

First, identify five things that you see in your immediate surroundings. Next, identify four things that you can reach nearby. Then, identify three things you can hear. Next, identify two things you can smell. Finally, identify one thing that you can taste.

DEBRIEF AND DIGEST

In this chapter, we covered five key lessons:

- There are a number of ways we can deal with challenging emotions such as anxiety, sadness, and anger.
- Emotional overwhelm can make us want to drink, but there are healthier ways for us to cope.
- When you want to run away from your difficult emotions, use CBT techniques to stand your ground.
- You can accept your feelings by inviting them in and cultivating self-compassion.
- Expressing ourselves in an assertive, healthy manner can help reduce our triggers that might otherwise lead to drinking in the long run.

SELF CHECK-IN

Find a comfortable seated or reclining position, close your eyes, and take a moment to reflect on how you are feeling. What emotions are you noticing? Where do you feel these emotions in your body?

Now take some time to reflect on what you read in this chapter. Did you learn anything new? Or were you reminded of some things that you have heard before? How do you think these tools could support your recovery?

I am powerful. I am forgiving.
I forgive myself for my past
actions and for harming
myself with alcohol. I can let
go and move forward.

Chapter 8

EMPOWER YOURSELF

Gaining a sense of empowerment is key to a successful life and a successful recovery. In this chapter, you will learn methods that will help you feel more empowered by boosting self-esteem, learning and practicing self-forgiveness, and letting go of any shame and guilt that may be surrounding your relationship to alcohol. Using these empowerment cultivating skills will help you create a more loving relationship with yourself, which will in turn support your recovery.

PRACTICING SELF-FORGIVENESS

After years of drinking in excess, you may be dealing with feelings of guilt and shame. You may feel guilty for the way you treated your body and your mind or ashamed for the way you treated other people when you were drunk. In order to move forward in recovery it is important that you address those feelings and work through letting them go. The act of self-forgiveness can be challenging for many people, but making an effort to forgive ourselves can empower us to let go of our pasts, feel relief in the present, and provide hope for the future.

Recognizing that we did not intend to hurt ourselves will help us soften around any harsh judgments that we have made of ourselves. In addition, acknowledging that we were doing the best we could at the time, with the coping tools that we had, will help us be more forgiving of ourselves. Lastly, reminding ourselves that we are not alone in being addicted to alcohol will help us feel more connected with others who have been through similar experiences, reducing any alienation that we may feel.

You Didn't Choose to Hurt Yourself

When you initially began drinking, your intention was not to hurt yourself. You may have been just drinking for fun, drinking to fit in, drinking to feel better, or drinking to self-medicate anxiety, stress, depression, or PTSD. At some point down the road, you may have realized that you were harming yourself by drinking; however, that knowledge isn't always enough motivation to quit on its own, especially for those of us who developed a dependency on alcohol. Recognizing that your initial intention when you started drinking was to take care of yourself can help reduce the feelings of shame and guilt associated with it and increase self-forgiveness.

You Did the Best You Could

For many people who struggle with alcohol-related issues, drinking serves as a coping skill for dealing with painful, uncomfortable emotions and social situations. Oftentimes, we do not have any other tools at our disposal to deal with these situations and feelings. Essentially, drinking often starts out as a way to meet your needs when you don't have any other skills. Acknowledging that you were doing the best that you could with what you knew/had at the time can help you soften the shameful feelings surrounding your alcoholism and learn to forgive yourself.

You Are Not Your Alcohol Addiction

Although you have had a difficult relationship with alcohol, your addiction does not define you. Being able to separate yourself from your alcohol dependence can be very empowering, helping you move forward in your recovery. When we separate ourselves from our addiction, we can see that we are more than our addiction, that we had worth before we started drinking, we had worth in the midst of our addiction, and we have worth in our recovery, no matter what our behaviors have been. There is more to us than our addictive behaviors, and that knowledge will help you separate yourself from identifying solely as an "addict" or "alcoholic."

FORGIVE YOURSELF

Although we can't change the past, we can change how we relate to it and to ourselves. Take a moment to reflect on some things you might be angry with yourself for, ways you have harmed or neglected yourself, or things you feel ashamed or guilty about. What would you like to forgive yourself for? What does it feel like to think about forgiving yourself?

_____

_____

_____

_____

_____

_____

_____

_____

_____

SELF-FORGIVENESS FOR YOUR BODY, HEART, AND MIND

The following exercise will help you forgive yourself for the way you have treated your body, heart, and mind.

Find a comfortable seated position. Sit up straight and close your eyes. Take a few deep breaths. Then place your hands on your body and say to yourself, "I forgive myself for the way I have treated my body." Take another breath and exhale out through the mouth. Put your hands over your heart and say to yourself, "I forgive myself for the way I have treated my heart." Take a deep breath and exhale out through the mouth. Put your hands on your head and say to yourself, "I forgive myself for the way I have treated my mind." Take a deep breath and exhale out through the mouth. Say to yourself, "I forgive you, I forgive you, I forgive you." Take one last deep breath and exhale out through the mouth, imagining you are exhaling all the built-up resentments, guilt, and shame you have been holding on to.

BUILD POSITIVE THINKING

After years of alcohol abuse, you may be accustomed to dwelling and ruminating on the negative emotions that come up, which can often feel overwhelming. For alcoholics, staying focused on negativity has a tendency to result in us reaching for a drink. Instead of constantly rehashing negative thoughts and emotions, you can learn how to cultivate and build up positive thinking by expanding and changing your perspective. In order to build positive thoughts, you must first come to realize that you have a choice in how you react to things. Another helpful skill in building positivity is to learn not to deny uncomfortable emotions, because doing so only strengthens them and can result in relapse. Lastly, practicing positive self-talk can aid in instilling a more optimistic mood as well as more self-confidence.

You Have a Choice in How You React

We may not always have much of a choice in the situations we find ourselves in; however, we do have a choice in how we react to them. Knowing that we have agency over our responses to situations, thoughts, and emotions can be quite empowering. Oftentimes, we get stuck on autopilot and aren't even aware of the way we're reacting, but we can break this kind of habitual behavior by taking a moment to pause, breathe, check in with ourselves, and make a conscious choice about how we move forward. For example, say your partner is late coming home from work. Your old response might be to jump to conclusions like "they're having an affair," or "they've been an accident," leading to anger or anxiety that might drive you to drink. But if you pause to think clearly, you might make a different choice about how you want to react.

Don't Deny Uncomfortable Emotions

Many of us may be in the habit of denying our uncomfortable emotions. This strategy, whether conscious or unconscious, may seem beneficial in the short term, but in the long term, choosing to ignore our emotions or deny that we have them can breed resentment and ultimately disconnect us from ourselves and others. Rather than denying our difficult feelings, we can learn ways in which we can come to accept them. Accepting our uncomfortable emotions can result in more connection with ourselves and others and can become a major tool for supporting our recovery.

Practice Positive Self-Talk

If we actually took the time to think about how much of our self-talk is negative and downright cruel, we would likely be astonished. Most of us talk negatively to ourselves throughout the day in ways that we would never speak to anyone else, especially someone we loved. So why not learn to talk to yourself in the way you would talk to someone you love? One way to do this is to ask yourself, "What would someone who loves themself say to themself in this situation?" We can learn to self-soothe by becoming aware of our internal dialogue and altering it to have a more supportive, positive emotional outcome.

BUILD SELF-LOVE AND POSITIVE THINKING

Take a moment to reflect on a few recent situations that caused you distress. What would someone who loves themself say to themself in that scenario? What would you say to someone you love who experienced something similar? Once you have written those things down, take a moment to reflect on how you feel. What emotions are you feeling now, and how have they changed since you started this exercise?

_____

_____

_____

_____

_____

_____

_____

BUILDING A POSITIVE PERSPECTIVE

Each day when you wake up, make a list of things that you are grateful for. It does not have to be a specific number of things, but if you need a number, aim for 10. The important part of this exercise is being able to tap into the feeling of appreciation and gratitude you have for the things that are already going well in your life. If you notice yourself getting into a negative headspace throughout the day, you can practice this exercise again. Make sure that you take time to close your eyes and really feel the feeling of appreciation in your body. After you do this exercise regularly for several days in row, notice if your perspective has shifted at all. By practicing gratitude regularly, we can train ourselves to see the world in a more positive light.

BUILD SELF-ESTEEM

After years of drinking to escape, or drinking to make yourself feel more desirable or interesting in social settings, you may be used to thinking less of yourself and not having much self-esteem or confidence when you are sober. Instead of drinking to cope with these issues, you can learn how to cultivate and build up self-esteem by expanding and changing your perspective.

In order to cultivate more positive thoughts about ourselves, we must first recognize that nobody is perfect and neither are we (or will we ever be). This will help reduce the expectation of being perfect that many people feel, and the shame that comes along with never achieving perfection, which can lead to drinking. Another way we can cultivate more positive thoughts is by celebrating small wins, which helps us recognize all the little things that we achieve along the way. And lastly, we can learn to reaffirm our own self-worth in order to cultivate more positivity. When we learn to practice and apply these beliefs and habits, our need to use alcohol as a crutch will lessen exponentially.

Nobody's Perfect

Many of us struggle to forgive ourselves for our past actions or our current dependency on alcohol because there is part of us that believes that we should already be perfect, and that we should be able to handle anything that comes our way. This is an example of black-and-white thinking, which we have already learned is not a realistic perspective (see page 58). Recognizing and accepting that nobody is perfect, including ourselves, can help us forgive and accept ourselves and our pasts as they are. This act of surrender will free us up to move forward while also improving our relationships with loved ones whom we can learn to grant the same generosity to.

Celebrate Small Wins

Many of us have a tendency not to recognize the small victories that we achieve, instead focusing on huge goals that feel impossible, which can lead to us feeling down on ourselves and believing we have already failed. Learning to acknowledge these small "wins" can help us develop more appreciation for ourselves and our accomplishments, thereby increasing our self-esteem. It's important to remember that large goals are always achieved as the result of a series of small achievements along the way.

Celebrating small wins is also important for maintaining a positive perspective in the face of setback. For instance, you may have gone a week without drinking and then have a drink. You may be upset with yourself for relapsing, but recalling the amount of time that you stayed sober before that drink can increase your self-esteem, granting you the confidence you need to maintain your sobriety even longer next time.

Reaffirm Your Self-Worth

After using alcohol to cope with emotions or provide a social lubricant, we may have conditioned ourselves to have low self-worth and believe that we cannot deal with these situations without alcohol. Reaffirming your innate self-worth can be another helpful way to increase self-esteem. It is important to remind yourself that no matter what, every human being has an innate self-worth—including you. We all have value and the potential for greatness when we apply ourselves. Consistently remind yourself of your self-worth by using affirmations and making lists of the things that you love about yourself and that other people love about you. It may take a little time, but eventually you will start to believe it.

RECOGNIZE YOUR ACCOMPLISHMENTS

Take a moment to reflect on what you have accomplished in the past month. Now make a list of the things you accomplished. Reflect on how it feels to have accomplished those things. Allow yourself to really sink into that feeling of accomplishment. How does it feel?

_____

_____

_____

_____

_____

_____

SELF-ESTEEM BOOST

Take some time to reflect on your self-worth. Find a comfortable seated position, close your eyes, and breathe. Place your hands on your heart. Connect with yourself. Think of some compliments that have been given to you by loved ones, employers, coworkers, teachers, or other important people in your life. Now think of some things that you love about yourself. Some examples of things that you may find redeeming about yourself could be an openness and willingness to try new things, determination to meet your goal of sobriety, or your ability to connect with your emotions and support other people. Breathe. When you are done, write that list down so you can refer back to it any time you need a reminder of your worth.

_____

_____

_____

_____

_____

_____

_____

DEBRIEF AND DIGEST

In this chapter, we covered five key lessons:
- You can feel more empowered by boosting your self-esteem, learning how to accept your past actions, and forgiving yourself.
- Letting go of shame and guilt that you may have acquired surrounding your alcohol addiction will create a more loving relationship with yourself, which will in turn support your recovery.
- You can learn to forgive yourself by recognizing your intentions, acknowledging that you are doing your best, and separating yourself from your addiction.

- You can boost your self-esteem by acknowledging your small wins, realizing that nobody is perfect, and affirming your innate self-worth.
- You can build a positive perspective by making conscious choices about your reactions, accepting your uncomfortable emotions, and practicing positive self-talk.

SELF CHECK-IN

Take some time to reflect on how you are feeling after completing this chapter. What emotions are you feeling? And where do you feel them in your body? Breathe.

Now take a moment to reflect on what you have read. Did you learn anything new? Is there anything that you feel resistant to? Is there anything you are excited to try?

_____

_____

_____

_____

_____

_____

_____

_____

_____

_____

_____

_____

_____

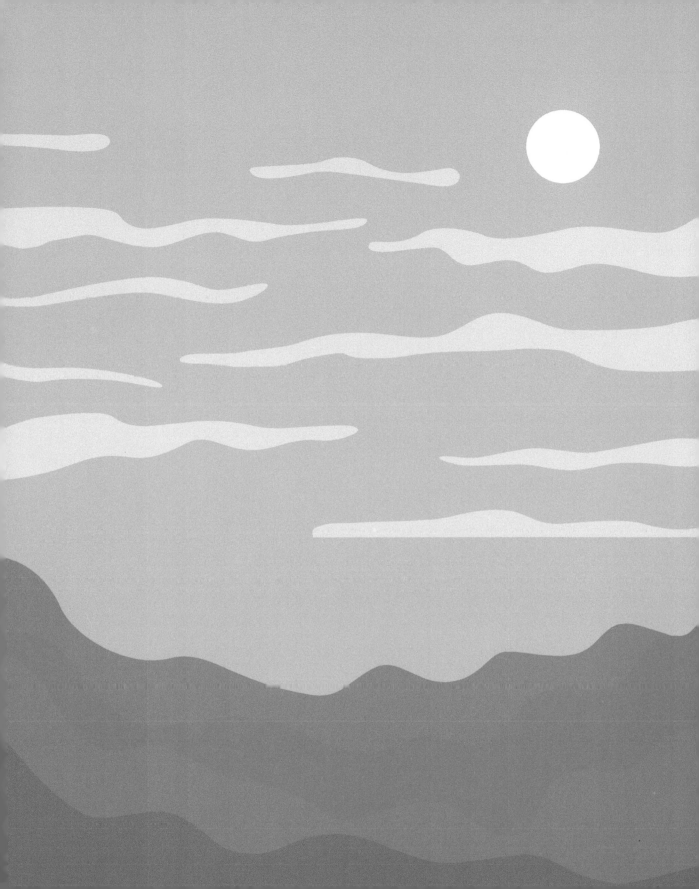

PART 3

STAYING SOBER

I can achieve my goals.
I can stay sober no matter what
happens. I never have to pick
up a drink again.

I can learn how to cultivate hope. I can let go. I am courageous. I can accept my past actions and the present situation and have hope for the future.

Chapter 9

BARRIERS TO RECOVERY

There are certain barriers to maintaining sobriety that can be a challenge for many alcoholics. In this chapter, we will discuss potential obstacles that may stand in the way of your recovery such as feeling hopeless, being afraid of letting go, being afraid of triggers that may lead you to drink, and the stigma surrounding alcoholism. We will also explore exercises and reflections that will help instill these concepts and create a working definition of them in your life.

FEELING HOPELESS

Clearly, losing hope can be detrimental to the recovery process. Many alcoholics in active addiction feel hopeless, but staying stuck in this feeling will likely cause them to also stay stuck in the vicious cycle of alcoholism. The good news is that we can counteract this sense of hopelessness by learning to cultivate small amounts of hope, which can accumulate and snowball into larger amounts. Powerful tools for cultivating hope are recognizing what we are grateful for, identifying what we have accomplished so far, and connecting with others who have been able to stay sober. Listening to other people's stories of struggle and how they overcame their struggles can be particularly powerful in supporting your recovery. Many 12-step recovery groups such as AA, Buddhist recovery groups like Recovery Dharma, and nonspiritual, CBT-oriented groups like SMART Recovery provide a community in which you can connect with others, hear their stories, and gain a sense of hope through their example and encouragement.

Anecdote

Many of us relapse quite a few times before we are able to maintain our sobriety long term. It is common to try and fail many times, to make and break many promises to ourselves, and it is easy to get discouraged and lose hope. I am one of those people for whom sobriety didn't take the first time. But I was able to break the cycle and gain hope by joining recovery communities, getting a sponsor, and befriending and reaching out to people in recovery communities. I found that being able to call sober people in recovery when I needed support was invaluable to my recovery. Also, hearing other people's stories in meetings helped me identify my own issues and provided me with the hope that I needed to keep going even when it was hard. Because other addicts who went through so many challenges were able to stay sober, I knew that I could, too.

HOPE THROUGH CONNECTION

Take a moment to think about who you know that is in recovery, is sober, or is supportive of your sobriety. Call three of those people, ask for their support, and ask them to share their story with you.

If you can't think of anyone that you can call, join a recovery or sobriety group on social media, make a post, and ask for the support of group members.

Another option is to find some sort of recovery meeting in person or online, group therapy, or an individual therapist who has experience working with alcoholism or other substance abuse. You can attend an AA meeting, a Buddhist recovery meeting, a SMART Recovery meeting, or another kind of recovery meeting. If those don't feel right, you can seek out a therapy group focused on alcoholism or substance use in general.

Reflection

Now take a moment to reflect on your own relationship with hope. Have you felt hopeless in the midst of trying to stay sober? Were you feeling hopeless before you started drinking in excess? How do you feel now after learning about some ways in which to cultivate hope?

FEAR OF LETTING GO

If you are struggling with quitting alcohol, it is likely that you are afraid to let go of it for a variety of reasons. You may fear not being able to use alcohol as a crutch, whether you are using it to bury or cope with difficult emotions or make social situations feel less anxiety provoking or more fun. You may lack confidence that you will be able to handle life's challenges without drinking, or you may be afraid of what feelings might surface if you remove the buffer of alcohol. You may be afraid of appearing like the odd one out in social settings by being the only one who does not drink. You may be accustomed to drinking in certain situations like at holidays, clubs, shows, parties, work events, happy hours, and bars. You may fear letting go of these social customs and opening yourself to new and perhaps vulnerable terrain. Staying sober can be a challenge when you are accustomed to alcohol being a part of so many facets of your life.

Anecdote

Sheila realized that the argument that we cannot have fun or be fun when we are sober is simply false. She noted that having fun while sober takes getting accustomed to, developing confidence in sobriety, and partaking in activities that feel fun to her in sobriety. Sheila realized that there are plenty of fun things to do without alcohol, and in fact, drinking actually limited her life.

Sheila attended social events like dances and parties hosted by recovery communities like AA. She found these events to be very helpful in supporting her desire to socialize without the temptations of alcohol. In early sobriety, Sheila found mindfulness and yoga tools to be particularly helpful in feeling comfortable with things like dancing. When she was feeling anxious or self-conscious in social situations, she made an effort to bring her focus to the people that she was with instead of how she felt others were perceiving her.

LET GO OF YOUR OLD WAYS

Make a list of some of things you'd like to do for fun without alcohol. Start small. Plan some friend dates or family time with the intention of being sober. You could go miniature golfing, bowling, hiking, or kayaking; make a nice meal; or go to an exercise class or a movie. Make it fun! The first few times may feel awkward, but soon enough you will become accustomed to living free of alcohol and you will see that having fun sober is totally doable if you have a positive mindset and are with fun, friendly people.

_____

_____

_____

_____

_____

_____

Reflection

Take a moment to reflect on any fears of letting go that you might have. What are you afraid of letting go of? What have you succeeded in letting go of in the past? What do you think it will take to let go of your drinking habit?

_____

_____

_____

_____

_____

_____

FEAR OF TRIGGERS

Another barrier to recovery for many women is having a fear of the triggers that have previously led them to drink. Some examples of potential triggers that you may fear and have drank over in the past are difficulties with a friend or partner, the death of a pet or loved one, stress at work, social anxiety, going on a date, taking a test or going to an interview, or experiencing thoughts and feelings that seem unbearable. Being afraid of how these events might feel without alcohol could lead you to drink even though you had set out to abstain from drinking. In the past we have resorted to alcohol to cope, so our brains are wired to go toward alcohol as a solution again and again. Breaking the habit of what we are accustomed to using to cope can be a challenge, but there are many tools that we have discussed in the previous chapters and will discuss in the following sections that can help with avoiding these pitfalls.

Some triggers to drink such as traumatic memories and PTSD may not feel safe to face alone. If you are feeling this way, please contact a mental health professional to help support you in this process.

Anecdote

Anna is a musician who used to fear playing live while she was sober, especially in front of her family. In fact, the last time she ever had a drink was before a performance that she was giving in front of her family members. She was so accustomed to performing under the influence that when she felt fear, her brain immediately went to the thought of drinking to cope with it. Eventually, Anna learned that she didn't have to drink for any reason or because of any feeling. She learned how to be more present in her body and use her breath and positive self-talk in order to overcome fear.

BUILDING COURAGE IN THE FACE OF TRIGGERS

When you are feeling stressed, anxious, or sad, you may be tempted to drink. Make a list of things that you can do to cope with those feelings that do not involve alcohol. Some examples of activities you could partake in are meditation, deep breathing, exercise, journaling, or reaching out to a supportive friend. Practice doing these activities when you are not feeling triggered so that you get in the habit of doing them. Then try doing some when you are feeling triggered and notice the difference after you engage in the activity. Write down the effect that the activity had on you.

Reflection

Think of some situations that have triggered you to want to drink in the past. What happened and what emotions were you feeling? How do you think you can deal with those triggers without alcohol? Perhaps name some of the tools and exercises that we have reviewed in previous chapters.

_____

_____

_____

_____

_____

_____

_____

THE STIGMA

The stigma surrounding alcohol dependence and sobriety can act as another barrier in recovery. Many people often frown upon those who drink in excess for a variety of reasons, including their religion, beliefs, or morals or due to them disapproving of the behaviors that tend to come along with excessive alcohol consumption. Some of the behaviors of people who overconsume alcohol might be the tendency to get angry, loud, violent, inconsiderate, or belligerent. Drinking in excess is also associated with increased risky behaviors when it comes to sex and could lower inhibitions around other behaviors like driving under the influence, consuming drugs, or committing crimes.

Ironically, there is also a stigma when it comes to sobriety. Drinking is so ingrained in our culture that people often look at sober people as though we are odd. We may get looked at as though we are too healthy, not fun, "square," too picky, etc. We may get left out or disinvited from social events because people who drink feel uncomfortable being around people who don't drink. Luckily, there is increasing mainstream acceptance of people who choose sober lifestyles. More and more people, including those who don't have a problem with alcohol, are prioritizing their physical, mental, and emotional health and opting out of drinking.

Anecdote

Tina often felt left out of social situations due to the fact that she was abstaining from alcohol. She realized that some people assumed that because she was sober that she didn't want to go to a bar or a club; however, she felt comfortable with this after many years of being sober. Tina found that when she felt secure in her sobriety and confident in her ability to implement tools to deal with triggers, she felt more comfortable attending events that serve alcohol.

Tina realized that people who have active drinking habits are likely to feel self-conscious about them when they are around someone who is sober. In these cases, Tina found it helpful to have open conversations with her friends about this and/or spend less time with friends who are avid drinkers. Tina found it very helpful to find sober friends, whether they were in recovery or were "straight edge" and never really drank much at all. She was surprised to discover that most people were actually very supportive of her decision to stop drinking, and the people who weren't were usually people who had drinking problems themselves.

DESTIGMATIZE YOUR LIFE

One way we can contribute to destigmatizing alcoholism and sobriety is by talking openly about it with friends and family and perhaps share on social media if it feels safe to do so. Addictions are quite common in today's culture, and it's encouraging to see so many people, including celebrities, talking more openly about their struggles and recovery. The less we hide them and the more we are open about them will contribute to the growing destigmatization. Personally, I feel like it is pretty "cool" to be sober in a culture where substance use is the norm. It means I have self-control and willpower, I have worked on myself, and I am choosing to prioritize my physical, mental, and emotional health. In fact, the more I hang out with sober or straight-edge people, the more I notice a growing stigma surrounding excessive alcohol consumption, and the more pride I feel in choosing to abstain from alcohol.

Take some time to make a list of ideas about ways in which you might want to be open about your sobriety. Who would you want to be open with, and what would you want to tell them?

Reflection

How has the stigma of alcoholism and recovery affected you? Do you think you might be further along in your recovery journey if it weren't for the stigma associated with sobriety or alcoholism? Do you think you may have sought treatment or support sooner? How do you think you can help destigmatize addiction and recovery/sobriety?

DEBRIEF AND DIGEST

In this chapter, we covered five key lessons:

- Recognizing what we are grateful for, identifying what we have accomplished so far, and connecting with others who have been able to stay sober are powerful tools for cultivating hope.
- Having fun sober is totally doable if you have a positive mindset and are with fun, friendly, and supportive people.
- Being afraid of triggers like anxiety, insecurity, stress, and sadness can lead us to drink, but engaging in new activities and coping strategies that do not involve alcohol builds courage.
- The stigma surrounding alcoholism and sobriety can be a barrier to maintaining sobriety, but more and more people are prioritizing their physical, mental, and emotional health and opting out of drinking.
- There are many obstacles that you may come across on the road toward maintaining your sobriety, but you have the tools and strategies to overcome them.

SELF CHECK-IN

Take a moment to reflect on how you are feeling after reading and completing the exercises in this chapter. What emotions are you feeling? Are you able to locate where you feel them in your body?

Now take a moment to reflect on what you learned from this chapter. Did you feel like you could relate to anything that was discussed in this chapter? Which parts?

_____

_____

_____

_____

_____

_____

I am strong. I am brave.
I can break habits and
go against the grain.
I can have fun and be fun
without alcohol.
I can change.

Chapter 10

ALCOHOL FREE WITH FRIENDS

Many alcoholics find it challenging to be in various types of social situations without having a drink. In this chapter, we will address how to let go of drinking in social settings. We will discuss bars and whether to ditch them, build our own plans for developing healthy habits, explore myths about drinking and alcohol dependence, and create strategies for maintaining a sober lifestyle. Lastly, we will complete exercises that will support us in being alcohol free in social situations.

DITCH THE BAR

Adjusting to a different type of social life can be a challenge for those who are attempting to quit drinking. Many people are hung up on going to bars in order to spend time with friends or meet new people. In fact, for many friendships, going to bars can represent the crux of the relationship. In this section we will discuss why bars are often seen as central to developing friendships, cultural pressures, and the alcohol industry, and harsh truths about social lives and alcohol.

Why Are Bars Central to Developing Friendship?

Many people find that in their adult lives, post high school or post college, it tends to be more difficult to make friends. Bars are seen as social events in themselves, because many people go to them several nights a week, and especially on weekends. For many, alcohol acts as a social lubricant and a way to bond with friends, acquaintances, coworkers, classmates, and strangers. A study on alcohol and group formation showed that drinking tends to increase social bonding when groups are formed. Unfortunately, you may find that friendships that were developed in bars may not last once you make a commitment to staying sober, because people who drink sometimes feel uncomfortable being around someone who doesn't drink. In addition, many people who are attempting to stay sober will feel uncomfortable being at bars and around people who are drinking, and this kind of environment may trigger a relapse. In recovery, it often becomes necessary to let go of this dependence on making friends and socializing at bars. Instead, we can make friends by engaging in activities that do not involve alcohol like going to in-person meetups or exercise classes or by volunteering, and we can socialize with existing friends by going out for coffee or doing activities that don't involve alcohol.

Cultural Pressures and the Alcohol Industry

Some additional difficulties that people in recovery may come upon are the cultural pressures to drink, as well as the push to drink by the alcohol industry. For many holidays it is considered tradition to drink and to drink in excess. In the United States, the most drinking during the year tends to occur in the time between Thanksgiving, Christmas, and New Year's Eve. The Fourth of July is another time when people tend to drink a lot. Police officers are on alert at these times of year because the alcohol consumption is seen as a threat to public health. On these holidays we may drink more because we feel pressured or stressed due to our family situations, cultural customs, as well as advertising encouraging alcohol consumption. For instance, many alcohol ads marketed to women suggest that women can bond with one another over alcoholic beverages.

Harsh Truths about Social Lives and Alcohol

It's likely that quitting drinking is going to significantly change your social life. You may find that the friendships that you made while drinking were sustained by your mutual interest in drinking, and once you quit alcohol, the friendship does not last. This harsh reality can be challenging for many people who want to quit drinking, but the upside is that you can make new friends you connect with based on mutual interests, not the substances that you ingest. Also, you can make friends with people who are in recovery as well and build strong bonds with them based on your similar past experiences. You may find that your relationships in sobriety have a stronger glue to them in general than your relationships that came out of drinking.

FRIEND OR FOE?

Take some time to reflect on your relationship with alcohol. How has your relationship with it impacted your life, particularly your relationships? In general, has your relationship with alcohol been more helpful or harmful? In your life, what are the pros and cons of drinking?

_____

_____

_____

_____

_____

_____

BUILD YOUR OWN PLAN

Loved ones, fellow recovery group members, therapists, and counselors may have many useful suggestions to help you maintain your sobriety; however, building your own plan is an important part of making it stick. Tailoring lifestyle changes and healthy habits specific to you and your recovery will make your plan more relevant and meaningful to you, and it will help you feel empowered on your sobriety journey. Some things you may want to include in your plan are lifestyle changes, long-lasting changes, and consideration of biological, emotional, and physical benefits.

Lifestyle Changes

What changes in your lifestyle do you think will support your journey to sobriety? For some people, this might look like avoiding clubs, bars, and potentially other places where alcohol is served for the time being or indefinitely. It may also mean taking a good look at your relationships and considering who you want to spend time with based on how supportive they will be of your decision to quit drinking. Involving stress-relieving activities like regular exercise, yoga, meditation, breathing exercises, and massage could be another positive lifestyle change that would support your goals. Lastly, eating healthy and ensuring that you have a regular sleep schedule, ideally going to bed by 10 p.m., can help support your mood and sobriety.

Long-Lasting Changes

Making long-lasting changes in your life is essential for staying sober. What are some long-term changes that you would like to make that could support your sobriety? Ideally, we would want to make changes that will support us physiologically, mentally, emotionally, spiritually, environmentally, and socially. Some ideas could be changing your diet to incorporate more nutritious foods; creating a regular exercise routine; starting a consistent mindfulness practice; joining a recovery community like AA, Recovery Dharma, or SMART Recovery; or getting into individual and/or group therapy. You can make a list of the changes that you would like to make, write out your long-term goals, and set a target date for when you would like to achieve them by.

Biological Benefits

To stay motivated on your recovery journey, it can be helpful to keep in mind the many biological benefits of maintaining sobriety. Many people find that when they stop drinking they feel better in general, sleep better, and think more clearly. In addition, when you quit drinking, you will have a reduced risk of heart complications such as high blood pressure, stroke, arrhythmia, and cardiomyopathy. You will also have reduced risk of pancreatitis, cancer, and liver complications like fatty liver, cirrhosis, fibrosis, and alcoholic hepatitis. Lastly, your immune system will strengthen and you will be less likely to develop pneumonia, tuberculosis, and infections.

Emotional Benefits

What are some of the emotional benefits of maintaining sobriety? Although many people use alcohol to self-medicate their mental health symptoms, research shows alcohol can actually worsen mental health symptoms. Therefore, when you stop drinking, it is likely that you will notice an improved sense of emotional well-being. A recent study found that women in particular are likely to experience improved mental health in long-term sobriety. The longer you stick with sobriety, the more you will see these emotional benefits. Not only is it likely that you will develop more confidence and self-respect, but it's also common to feel less depression and anxiety after quitting alcohol. By not using alcohol to run from or numb uncomfortable feelings, you are more likely to be able to access the awareness and resolve to heal emotional wounds.

Physical Benefits

What are some of the physical benefits of maintaining sobriety? Many people find that they look better and younger after abstaining from drinking for a while. Those who quit alcohol often observe that their faces appear healthier and more attractive, especially their skin. Because alcohol is a diuretic, causing your skin to lose elasticity and dehydrating you, you will naturally become more hydrated and your collagen will normalize when you stop drinking. In addition, you may lose weight, because when we drink in excess, we are often consuming extra calories that can lead to weight gain. You will also notice improvements in sleep and increased energy.

CHANGE HABITS, CHANGE YOUR BRAIN

When you change your habits, you are essentially changing your brain. Even though it feels impossible now, it is entirely within your control to change your lifestyle, build new, healthier habits, and decrease the role that alcohol plays in your life. We all have the ability to change.

Dopamine Hit

Dopamine is a neurotransmitter in the brain that transports important messages. It serves many functions and is connected with reward-seeking behavior, motivation, craving, addiction, and drug dependency. According to research, even the smallest taste of certain types of alcohol can lead us to consume more because the brain reacts with a flood of dopamine.

Learning to engage in other behaviors and activities that increase dopamine levels can support us in our sobriety. We can essentially retrain the reward centers in our brain to get activated by behavior besides drinking. There are many ways that you can increase levels of dopamine in your brain, including exercising frequently, getting adequate sleep, listening to music, meditating, getting adequate sun exposure, and ensuring that you are getting enough vitamins and minerals like niacin, iron, vitamin B6, and folate.

Neuroplasticity

Scientists used to believe that brain damage was irreversible; however, neuroscientists have more recently disproved this theory. Although some neurons may be permanently damaged, the brain is able to heal itself by creating new neural pathways. This process is known as *neuroplasticity*, or in other words, brain or neuron moldability. Alcoholism can be considered a neuroplastic event, because over time the brain becomes conditioned to drink. But that also means that the brain can be reconditioned to *not* drink. With various forms of treatment such as mindfulness, CBT, and trauma-focused treatments like eye movement desensitization reprocessing (EMDR), you can retrain the brain to develop new neural pathways that will help you maintain your sobriety.

Strategies for Breaking Habits

Not only is compulsive drinking a habit we want to break, but when we are addicted to a drug like alcohol, we oftentimes have developed a variety of other bad habits as well—like not giving our body the nutrition it needs, not getting enough sleep, not exercising, and not keeping our spaces clean or our appearances up. In fact, in recovery communities it is common for sponsors to suggest that their sponsees make their bed every morning when they wake up, or to call every day to create the habit of reaching out for help. Some additional ways to break habits are creating reminders for yourself, replacing habits with different ones, starting small, changing your surroundings, practicing self-care, and being patient with yourself.

Strategy #1

Create reminders. You can create reminders by entering appointments into a physical calendar or a phone calendar. There you can keep track of any recovery meetings or therapy appointments, schedule your exercise and mindfulness routines, and schedule any calls you may want to make to supportive people or sober friends.

Strategy #2

Replace harmful habits with healthier ones. If you are accustomed to drinking when you feel anxious, try a breathing technique instead. If you tend to drink when you come home from work, try practicing yoga, taking a long walk, or going to a recovery meeting instead. If you're used to reaching for a drink when you feel sad, reach for your phone instead and call or text a friend.

Strategy #3

Start out with small goals, like meditating for 5 minutes every morning, and as time moves on, increase it to 10 or 15 minutes. Start with a short walk around the neighborhood, then maybe increase the distance a little every few days. Congratulate yourself each time you meet your small goal.

BREAK YOUR HABITS, CHANGE YOUR BRAIN

Take a few minutes to enter a few recovery-related things that you would like to do into your calendar. You can schedule the time that you would like to work on this book, any recovery meetings that you would like to attend, or daily meditation or exercise times. Set reminders and start small. If you stick with them long enough, eventually these changes will become habit. Remember not to beat yourself up when you don't do everything perfectly. If you miss something one day, make a commitment to start again and do it tomorrow.

THE SOBRIETY ETHOS

In order to fully let go of drinking, it is necessary to also work on letting go of a few myths and fallacies, such as "Everyone can drink in moderation," "Drunk words are sober thoughts," "I don't drink as much as my friends," and "I can't be an alcoholic because . . ." Adopting a sobriety ethos, or a set of values and practices, will support you in your recovery. Gaining an understanding of the fallacies about drinking and the truth behind these common myths will help you embrace the idea of sobriety.

Myth: Everyone Can Drink in Moderation

Many people swear by the idea of "everything in moderation," meaning that people can imbibe in any vice as long as they don't overdo it, which can be a wise approach to life in many instances. However, for most addicts and alcoholics, the abstinence approach appears to be much more effective, as many of us learn the hard way when we try to moderate our alcohol use. It is common for people with drinking problems to try many ways to moderate or control their use, such as making rules about when and where and how much they can drink, but many of us find that these attempts ultimately fail. We pay the price of attempting to cut down without fully quitting with physical illness, relationship issues, DUIs, job losses, overdoses, and jail time. Although it may seem tempting to attempt moderating our drinking, unfortunately many of us are not able to meet this feat and realize eventually that we cannot drink like "normal" people. In AA literature, one of the signs of an alcoholic is someone who has attempted to moderate their drinking but has been unable to do so.

Myth: Drunk Words Are Sober Thoughts

Alcohol is well known for lowering inhibitions, which can lead us to engage in risky behaviors like unprotected sex, driving drunk, or behaviors that may cause social conflict like oversharing or inappropriate speech. Although many people believe that what we say when we are drunk is what we are thinking when we are sober, there is no research to support this theory. Alcohol is not a truth serum, and people certainly do not always tell the truth when they are under the influence of alcohol. So, if we are looking to alcohol to help ourselves have a difficult conversation, we may want to think twice about it, because it could turn out that we say things we don't mean or aren't actually true.

Myth: I Don't Drink as Much as My Friends

Many of us who may question whether we have a problem with alcohol will look at our friends' or significant other's drinking habits and feel that our problem pales in comparison to theirs. It is common for people to use the fact that their relationship with alcohol is not as much of a problem as their loved one's as a way to justify or minimize their own dependence on drinking. The truth is, many of us who drink in excess surround ourselves with others who also drink in excess, so the comparison might not be an accurate representation of a "normal" or healthy relationship to alcohol. But most importantly, what matters is your *own* relationship to alcohol. What are the pros and cons of drinking *for you*? Is it bad enough *for you*?

Myth: I Can't Be an Alcoholic Because . . .

The behavior of an alcoholic is not necessarily one size fits all. The classic idea of an alcoholic is someone who drinks all day long from morning to night, cannot sustain a job, and is physically addicted to alcohol. There are many other types that can fit into the definition of an alcoholic—like those who binge drink on occasion, those who drink in excess on the weekends, and "functional alcoholics" who can hold down a job or go to school while they maintain their alcohol addiction. This myth prevents many people from realizing or admitting that they may have a problem with alcohol.

EXPLORING MODERATION

Many of us have tried to moderate our alcohol consumption many times before coming to the decision that we need to abstain entirely. Reflect on some of the ways that you have tried to control or manage your drinking in the past that didn't work.

Many of us have not been honest with ourselves about the impact that our relationship with alcohol has had on our lives. We may have had difficulty admitting that we have a problem or have even lied to ourselves about it. Can you relate to this, and if so, what are some of the ways that you have not been honest with yourself about your relationship with alcohol?

STRATEGIES FOR A SOBER SOCIAL LIFE

Laying out a strategy for a sober social life will help ensure your success in recovery. You can learn to embrace your social life outside of the old habits that harmed you by planning ahead, reconnecting with your body, practicing meditation, and having a plan in case you relapse.

Plan Ahead

Making a plan ahead of time for how you will deal with certain circumstances when you come across them will support you in your recovery. For instance, what would you do if a friend or family member were to bring alcohol to your house? Or what would you do if you were at a social event that suddenly started serving alcohol? It is up to you to decide what your comfort level is in these situations and to set boundaries and make decisions accordingly. Many people who are in recovery prefer not to have alcohol in their homes and try to avoid venues where alcohol is served. If you are being completely honest with yourself, what are you comfortable with? What tools and resources can you have in your back pocket to help you respond wisely to challenges that come up?

Reconnect with Your Body

Connecting with our bodies can help us get out of our heads, enter into the present moment, and reduce uncomfortable feelings that may result in drinking. Making a habit of reconnecting with your body throughout the day can help you maintain your sobriety. Try going out for a walk, lifting weights, practicing yoga, dancing, or simply closing your eyes and focusing on what is going on in your body at the moment. If you are familiar with yoga, doing a few full, half, or quarter sun salutes can effectively help you reconnect with your body and breath.

Practice Meditation: Slow Down and Sit with Your Feelings

As mentioned throughout this book, another powerful strategy for maintaining a sober social life is practicing meditation. When we meditate, we are essentially taking time to slow down and ground ourselves, which can help reduce any anxiety we may feel in social situations. Studies have also shown that long-term meditation produces neuroplastic effects, essentially rewiring the brain for increased attention, self-regulation, and sensory processing. In meditation, we can practice "sitting with our feelings," or focusing on them and sending them awareness and compassion. Sitting with our feelings can oftentimes result in them dissipating or losing the power they held over us before we began our meditation practice. Nowadays, many of us have access to great meditation apps on our phones and meditation videos on the internet. There are also in-person meditation groups or "sanghas" you can look into joining. You can also use a script from a book or simply focus on your breath and body.

Alcohol Recovery: If You Drink, Return to Your Plan

In AA and other recovery communities, it is common for people to say that relapse is part of recovery. Although we may not want to imagine ourselves relapsing, it is important to have a plan in case we do relapse. Our plan could involve reaching out to a sober or supportive friend, a member of a recovery community, or a therapist. We may also want to begin attending some type of recovery meetings, psychotherapy group, and/or meditation groups. The key to getting back to sobriety after relapse is self-forgiveness, compassion, and cultivating hope. There are many self-forgiveness meditations available on video channels such as YouTube or meditation apps like Insight Timer. If prayer is part of a spiritual practice for you, you can also practice a self-forgiveness prayer if you like. Hope can be cultivated by connecting with people that I mentioned earlier and also reminding yourself of how far you've come. Make sure to reconnect with your "why" for getting sober, and you will be back on the path in no time!

In the Moment

The following exercise will help you manage/alleviate the overwhelming feelings that may occur as you work through this book and the prompts. This will help you learn how to manage your emotions over time and provide you with a way to address any urges you may have to drink when they arise. More specifically, this simple exercise will help you cultivate more compassion for yourself.

Find a comfortable seated position on a cushion or on a chair. Sit up with a straight spine, start to notice your breath, and become aware of your body. Notice your feet on the floor, get a sense of your arms and legs, and fully inhabit your body here. Take a few minutes to connect with your breath. Now bring to mind something that you have been criticizing yourself for lately, perhaps something that makes you feel that you are not enough. Notice how you feel when you think about this. Do you notice any tension in the face, the shoulders? Connect with your heart and notice how it feels when you think about your imperfection. Now say to yourself, "May I be peaceful, may I be kind to myself, may I be safe, and may I accept myself as I am." Repeat these phrases silently to yourself for a few minutes. Then take a moment to observe how you feel physically and emotionally.

DEBRIEF AND DIGEST

In this chapter, we covered five key lessons:

- Evaluating your relationship to alcohol involves evaluating your personal relationships. Changes to how and with whom you socialize will likely be necessary.
- You can learn to embrace your social life outside of the old habits that harmed you by practicing meditation and reconnecting with your body.
- Gaining an understanding of the fallacies about drinking and the truth behind common myths will help you embrace the idea of sobriety.

- Creating and sticking to a plan for how you are going to maintain your sobriety and cope with potential relapse will help keep your progress steady.
- Light yoga exercise can help you cope with overwhelm and get more grounded in your body and the present moment.

SELF CHECK-IN

Take a moment to reflect on how you're feeling emotionally. What feelings came up for you while reading this chapter and completing the exercises? Where do you feel those feelings in your body and what do they feel like?

Now take a moment to reflect on what you've learned in this chapter. What sticks out to you? How can you use this knowledge on your path to recovery?

I can learn. I can relax.
I can try new things.
I can let go of thoughts
about alcohol and focus
on my well-being. I can
overcome challenges.

Chapter 11

CHOOSE YOUR PATH

In the upcoming chapter, we will discuss some mindful relaxation techniques that you can add to your collection of healthy coping tools, like deep relaxation, progressive muscle relaxation, visualization, and learning to redirect your focus toward yourself and your overall well-being. We will also discuss how recovery is a journey, target some sobriety challenges, and identify strategies for growth and support systems.

THE RELAXATION APPROACH

Mindfulness is the practice of paying attention to the present moment, often using various points of focus like the breath, the body, visualization, and mantras. Mindfulness has been around as long as humans have existed; however, the formal practice of mindfulness is known to have been developed in India, when people there started to explore how they perceive things in a scientific manner while sitting near the Ganges and Indus Rivers.

Some studies show that using mindfulness practices can be an effective tool in addressing alcoholism. When we make it a practice to be aware of our thoughts and emotions, we can be more intentional about the choices we make in response to them, such as choosing a healthy coping tool rather than mindlessly reaching for a drink. Mindfulness practices make it possible to encourage your brain to send signals that tell it to slow down your muscles and organs and increase blood flow to the brain, thereby reducing stress and reactivity. Additionally, mindfulness practices can help us enter into our parasympathetic nervous system, also known as our rest and relaxation nervous system. The parasympathetic nervous system is essentially the opposite of the sympathetic nervous system, which is what drives our fight-or-flight response. When we are emotionally triggered with stress or anxiety, we are often in fight-or-flight mode, which can make it difficult to think clearly and make empowered choices. Using mindfulness to enter into our parasympathetic nervous system can help reduce the strength of our emotional triggers.

LEARNING TO RELAX

You can learn how to relax while sober by using your breath and your body and focusing your attention using mindfulness practices. Some ways that you can relax in a sober setting are by using deep relaxation techniques, muscle relaxation or progressive muscle relaxation, and visualization or guided imagery.

Deep Relaxation

This deep relaxation technique is great to practice when you come home from work, after you've been out, to unwind after a long day, or when you would like to relieve stress of any kind.

Lie down on your back in a quiet, dark, or dimly lit room. Put a pillow under your head. You can also place a pillow under your knees if you would like. This can especially help if your lower back feels tight. Close your eyes and take long, smooth breaths. Scan your body from head to toe, softening each area as you observe. Start with observing how your head feels, your face, eyes, nose, and lips. Then move on to observing your neck and throat, chest, arms, and hands, back and stomach, genital area and buttocks, and then your legs and feet. Spend several minutes observing your body. Notice how you feel afterward. Has anything changed?

Muscle Relaxation/Progressive Muscle Relaxation

Find a comfortable, quiet place where you can lie down. Now we will go through a variety of muscle groups in the body and you will be asked to tense them. Tense the muscles tightly, but not in a way that causes pain, for 4 to 10 seconds. Then, immediately and fully release your muscles, relaxing and observing the difference between clenching and relaxation for 10 to 20 seconds.

On an inhale, clench your hands tightly. Now extend the wrists and forearms, bending your hands back at the wrist. Now make fists with your hands, bend your arms at the elbows, and flex your biceps.

Raise your shoulders up to your ears. Wrinkle your forehead while frowning. Close your eyes tightly.

Smile as wide as possible. Press your lips together as tight as you can without tensing other parts of your face. Press your head against the floor.

Draw your chin toward your chest without tensing your head and neck. Inhale deeply, then hold, let go, relax, and observe how it feels to have released.

Arch your back. Suck your stomach in. Tense your buttocks. Clench your thighs. Flex your toes, then point them.

Now let all of that tension go and relax your body completely. Lie in stillness for as long as you need to enjoy this deep relaxation.

Visualization and Guided Imagery

Find a comfortable seated position. Close your eyes and take a few full, deep breaths. Bring a place to mind that brings you a sense of peace, calm, or joy. Imagine what it looks, smells, feels, tastes, and sounds like. Immerse yourself in that place for 5 to 10 minutes, gently noticing whatever sensory details arise. Then shift your attention to your body. How do you feel in this place, in this moment?

FOCUS ON YOURSELF

Learning how to focus on your well-being rather than focusing on when you are going to have your next drink will support your recovery significantly. Your days have most likely been dominated by thinking about drinking. Because of this, you probably have not been focusing on your well-being, and you may have even been neglecting some of your basic needs like nutrition, hydration, and sleep. In order to make the switch to focusing on your wellness, it's necessary to examine and create new daily habits and practices. In the sections to follow, I will provide mindful approaches to improving your sleep, nourishment, exercise habits, and relationships.

Sleep

Many people who are dependent on alcohol struggle with sleep and cite long-term improvements when they stop drinking. It is common for people in general to struggle with sleep issues such as difficulty falling asleep, waking up in the middle of the night and having trouble going back to sleep, waking up too early, and getting quality sleep. How well we sleep has a huge effect on our emotional and physical well-being. Not getting enough sleep can also negatively impact your work, your relationships, and your family. Insomnia that is short term, or lasting less than three weeks, can often be helped by common sleep hygiene techniques like exercising regularly, avoiding prolonged exposure to electronic screens (especially before bed), taking a hot shower or bath, or listening to soothing sleep soundtracks. If you have had difficulty sleeping for over three weeks, you may want to see your physician and/or a sleep doctor to determine if there are any underlying issues such as sleep apnea, restless leg syndrome, REM sleep behavior disorder, insomnia, or narcolepsy.

There are a wide variety of options for treating sleep issues. In addition to cultivating good sleep habits such as a regular sleep schedule and avoiding anything stimulating before bed like screens and vigorous exercise, techniques that help you relax such as progressive muscle relaxation and mindfulness practices can be helpful. Medication is also an option; however, many people experience unpleasant side effects, and the medication approach is generally considered a temporary solution by doctors. Some people find that occasional use of supplements such as melatonin and valerian root are helpful, but these are not supported by research and are not FDA approved. If your thoughts are keeping you up at night, CBT can help you examine and reframe any thoughts that may keep you from sleeping, creating more soothing, sleep-inducing thoughts. Lastly, light therapy, which helps you adjust to your circadian rhythm by exposing you to artificial light, can help improve sleep.

Strategy #1

Make a habit of going to sleep early, by 10 p.m. ideally. If you struggle with going to sleep early, try going to bed 15 to 30 minutes earlier each night or every few nights until you have reached the time that you would like to fall asleep. You can also use sleep hygiene techniques to encourage yourself to go to bed earlier like sleeping in a dark, comfortable, and quiet place, taking a hot shower or bath, and exercising during the day.

Strategy #2

Try to go to sleep at the same time every night and wake up at the same time every morning. Try to avoid taking long naps during the day. Having a regular sleep schedule can improve quality of sleep and help regulate emotions.

Strategy #3

Stay away from screens for an hour before bed and put your phone in a room other than the one that you are sleeping in. Being on our phone, computer, or other technological device can cause us to become stimulated, which can disrupt our ability to fall asleep. Reading a book in bed for 15 to 30 minutes is an excellent activity to help you ease into sleep.

SLEEP ROUTINE

For a week, try to go to bed early, by 10 p.m. or so, and stay away from all screens from 9 p.m. until an hour after you wake up. Observe any differences in your emotional state.

Nourishment

The food and drink that we put into our bodies greatly impacts our emotional and physical health. Most people who are dependent on alcohol have neglected their nutrition, and often a significant portion of the calories that they consume is from alcohol—approximately 25 to 50 percent. Many alcoholics suffer from health problems that are related to poor nutrition such as high blood pressure, high cholesterol, type 2 diabetes, and liver complications. Instead of focusing on alcohol, focusing on improving your health through consuming nutritious foods can greatly support your recovery. Adding a wide variety of fresh fruits and vegetables to the diet can help reduce sodium intake, which can lower blood pressure and also lower fat intake, which helps with lowering cholesterol. Fresh fruit and vegetable intake also significantly contributes to our level of hydration. Because alcohol is a diuretic, pulling fluids from our body, drinking leads to dehydration, especially if not enough water or water-rich produce is consumed. Therefore, consuming water-rich produce can reverse the dehydrating effect of alcohol. In addition, although there is more research needed to support the connection between blood sugar levels and mental health, some research suggests that reducing refined sugars and increasing complex carbohydrates and protein can help regulate blood sugar and thereby regulate mood.

Why fresh (or raw) fruits and vegetables? A study showed that cooking fruits and vegetables reduces some of their benefit to our mental health, whereas consuming them raw showed higher levels of mental health. The foods that were particularly effective at reducing depression were kiwi, bananas, cucumber, berries, citrus fruits, dark leafy greens, apples, and carrots. In addition to consuming an abundance of fresh fruits and vegetables, avoiding fast food and processed foods that come in packages, such as soda, chips, candy, and frozen meals, may also help in reducing depression.

Strategy #1

Try to shop mostly in the outer sections of the grocery store, which is where you will usually find the most nutritious foods such as fresh produce, eggs, and, if you eat meat, lean meats. Avoid the inner aisles in the grocery store that contain soda, candy, chips, frozen meals, and other processed foods.

Strategy #2

Eat an abundance of fresh fruits and vegetables, at least 5 to 9 servings a day according to the USDA. Making smoothies can be an excellent way to pack a lot of fruits and vegetables into your diet.

Strategy #3

Buy a new health promoting cookbook or experiment with healthy recipes you find online.

CREATING A FOOD PLAN

Creating a food plan and doing food prep for the week can make it a lot easier to eat healthy. Make a list of the meals that you would like to prepare for the week and their ingredients and go shopping for them. Schedule a time when you can food prep for the week. Many people find that Sunday is a good day to food prep because it is the day before the start of the workweek. If you prefer to eat freshly prepared meals every day, you can also just purchase any ingredients you need for the week or for the next few days and prepare the meal just before eating it or in the morning or evening before work. Fresh fruit, smoothies, and salads can be particularly simple to prepare in this case.

Exercise

Most people are aware that exercising regularly plays a significant role in supporting mental health. However, implementing an exercise routine can be a challenge for many, particularly those who are struggling with depression. How can we tackle this issue? Exploring various forms of exercise and identifying your favorite types;

committing to a regular exercise schedule, perhaps with a partner; attending a group exercise class; and practicing joyful movement can increase motivation to exercise. A study showed that exercise improved recovery rates for drug addicts who are attempting to maintain sobriety. The study emphasized the importance of behavioral change and the influence of peers to support long-term sobriety.

More research is needed in the area of exercise's impact on AUD. However, because exercise generally reduces stress and improves mental and physical health overall, it is reasonable to conclude that it supports efforts to maintain sobriety in the long term.

Strategy #1

Try a few different types of exercise like yoga, Pilates, dance, weight-lifting, spin class, bootcamp, martial arts, swimming, walking, hiking, or jogging. Have an open mind as you try each one, and pay attention to how you feel during and after. Remember, it can be helpful to start small. If you have not exercised in years, it would probably be wise to start with walking before attempting to run five miles. Having reasonable expectations and reachable goals will help ensure your success and likelihood of sticking with it.

Strategy #2

Pick the forms of exercise that you like the best and do them regularly, aiming for most days of the week. According to the CDC, a combination of 150 minutes of moderate aerobic exercise and two muscle strengthening workouts a week would be ideal. Again, it may take time for you to build up to this goal, and that's totally okay.

EXERCISE ROUTINE

Try many different types of exercise, perhaps a few different classes or solitary forms of exercise. Choose the ones that you enjoy the most and do them regularly. Aim to exercise nearly every day at the same time.

Relationships

Relationships can cause a good deal of stress, yet they can also provide a lot of support. Cultivating healthy relationships plays a significant role in maintaining your sobriety. First off, take some time to examine your relationships. Are your friends, family members, and/or significant other supportive of your sobriety? How would you characterize your relationships with them? Are these all people that you would like to keep in your life, that will be supportive of your sobriety?

Now think about the role that you have played in your relationships. Do you tend to hold your feelings in or do you communicate them? Do you ask for what you need or do you allow your needs to be swept under the rug? Are you able to say no or do you have people-pleasing tendencies? Many people who struggle with alcoholism also have difficulties with their relationships. Learning how to assertively communicate your feelings, express your needs, and set boundaries with the people in your life can provide a fruitful pathway on your road to recovery.

Strategy #1

Communicate your feelings. Instead of saying something like "You make me angry" to your loved one, use "I feel" statements such as "I feel angry when you raise your voice." Instead of "I hate when you talk to me that way!" say "I feel disrespected when you talk to me that way." Notice the difference in how your loved ones respond.

Strategy #2

Communicate your needs. Once you have expressed your feelings, you can ask for what you need. For example, you could say, "I would really appreciate it if you could speak to me in a respectful way." Women in particular are socialized to be people-pleasers, putting their needs second to everyone else's. This often builds resentment and loneliness that can lead us to drink. Communicating your needs can be an especially important tool for many women in recovery.

Strategy #3

Set boundaries. Learning to say no is one example of setting boundaries, which can be difficult for many people, especially women. If inside you want to say no, but you feel guilty, try saying something like "Unfortunately I'm not going to be able to do that," or you can ask for time to think about whether you will agree to meet their request. Remember that when you say yes to something, you are also usually saying no to something else; if the something else you're saying no to is yourself and your own needs, that may be a sign that you need to set some boundaries.

SHARING FEELINGS ASSERTIVELY

Take a moment to think about someone you may feel resentful of. Maybe you are angry or frustrated about something they did, or you feel like you aren't being heard or getting your needs met in the relationship. Now, think of what you may want to say to them. This could be something like "I feel disrespected when you leave a mess in the kitchen" or "I feel hurt when you cancel our plans at the last minute." How does it feel to think about saying that to someone? Now think of a few other situations and choose one to try communicating with someone.

DEFINE YOUR GROWTH

You, and only you, can define your own growth and recovery. Recovery is not a straight line but a journey with lots of curves and ups and downs. Although the road to sobriety may seem intimidating or complex, you can do it! You have the power to seek the support you need and change your routines. You can recover.

Your relationship with alcohol and your recovery from dependence on it impacts a wide variety of aspects of your life. You will notice that maintaining your sobriety will positively impact your relationships, your mental and physical health, your career, and your life goals in general. Sobriety is within your grasp. Your current or past relationship with alcohol and your emotions surrounding it does not need to determine how you live your life from this point forward. You don't have to remain feeling sad, hopeless, or disempowered. Because of the brave work you have done in this book, you now have a solid foundation of knowledge and resources to go forward and change your life. Although you may experience some twists and turns along the way, I know you can persevere and stay on track. Having gotten this far in this workbook shows that you are truly motivated to make change happen in your life. I wish you the best in your recovery!

GOAL SETTING

Make a list of some of your recovery-related goals and note when you would like to achieve them by and what steps you are going to take in order to get there.

GOAL	GOAL DATE	STEPS I'M GOING TO TAKE

TARGETED SOBRIETY CHALLENGES

In this section we will identify some triggers that may make staying sober difficult for you in the future, so you can be prepared with a plan to deal with them when they come up. Some categories of potential triggers that may make you want to drink could be emotional, environmental, and social triggers. In all of these situations, you can choose to walk away or take a break, and you can also use the CBT and mindfulness/relaxation skills that you have learned in the previous chapters. In time, using these skills will become second nature to you. You will feel prepared to deal with any situation and come to realize that with all of these tools available to you, you never have to drink again.

Emotional Triggers

Some examples of emotional triggers are feeling anxious due to an upcoming deadline, feeling depressed or lonely due to a lack of community or friendships, and feeling stressed from work or family. To cope with these triggers, you can use some of the CBT skills that we learned about earlier, such as the thought record. You can also use some of the mindfulness and relaxation skills like meditation, yoga, and progressive muscle relaxation. Reaching out and talking to a trusted friend can also be a great way to work through strong emotions. Many people find that various forms of exercise such as jogging, dancing or swimming can also be an effective way to cope with emotional triggers.

Environmental Triggers

You may find that you become triggered by your environment. Many people tend to drink at parties, club, bars, and holiday celebrations. You may want to avoid places or events where you used to drink while you are gaining strength in your sobriety. What time of day did you find yourself drinking the most? For instance, you may start drinking when you get home from work or late in the evening when you go out. Once you identify what times of the day you tend to drink, you can use that knowledge to be prepared with tools and activities to partake in at those times that don't involve alcohol.

Social Triggers

Social situations can be triggering for many people who are attempting to stay sober. Make a list of the people that you have drank with in the past and/or who may be triggering for you to be around. You may want to avoid spending time with these people when you're early in sobriety or indefinitely. If you choose to spend time with them, it would be a good idea to inform them of your sobriety goals and request that they do not bring alcohol around you. When you feel triggered, you may also want to consider walking away, taking a break, contacting a supportive friend or a recovery community member, taking deep breaths, and reminding yourself that you don't have to drink over anything.

STRATEGIES FOR GROWTH

Developing a sustainable "maintenance" program can help you maintain your sobriety and support your growth. Some strategies that you can use to support your sobriety and fuel your growth are starting a journal, avoiding social functions that involve alcohol, focusing on joyful movement, being mindful of your social media use, and developing a regular mindfulness practice.

Strategy #1: Start a Journal

Get a journal or notebook to carefully monitor your feelings, behaviors, and impulses that might lead to wanting to have a drink. Monitoring will allow you to understand and identify the precise factors that are triggering your drinking behavior. You can also use your journal to express and process your feelings instead of reaching for a drink.

Strategy #2: Avoid Functions with Alcohol

You may want to avoid social functions that involve alcohol for the time being or indefinitely in order to reduce the temptation to drink. Some places that you may want to avoid are bars, clubs, and parties where alcohol is served. You can replace these alcohol-focused events with healthier activities like hiking, exercise classes, sober dinner parties, going to the park, shopping, and meeting at coffee or juice shops.

Strategy #3: Focus on Joyful Movement

Getting into your body can help you get out of your head, and focusing on joyful movement can bring more joy into your life! If you weren't thinking about having a drink, what could you be doing to bring mindful, joyful movement into your life? Get an exercise mat and put it on the floor, listen to your body, and begin moving in ways that feel good to you. You can put on music and dance or do stretching or yoga if you like.

Strategy #4: Be Mindful of Your Social Media Use

Many people find that limiting social media helps support their mental health and personal growth. Although some of my clients have found it helpful to limit social media due to the anxiety, comparisons, and FOMO (fear of missing out) that it can produce, others have found that following recovery and sobriety hashtags and participating in online sobriety/recovery groups have been supportive of their journey. The key is making intentional, mindful choices based on what is best for you. You may want to unfollow certain influencers or friends on social media that trigger you to feel anxious or depressed; however, you may find that following accounts that inspire you can be helpful. Either way, limiting time on social media can help you focus on your own life, goals, and dreams.

Strategy #5: Develop a Regular Mindfulness Practice

In the previous chapters we identified a variety of mindfulness practices such as meditation, deep relaxation, yoga, tai chi, breathwork, and progressive muscle relaxation, which can all support you in your growth. Developing a consistent mindfulness practice can be particularly helpful. Try doing a mindfulness practice every morning for at least 5 to10 minutes. You can try using mindfulness apps that provide lots of guided meditations like Calm, Headspace, and Waking Up. Starting out the day in a mindful way will inevitably lead to emotional growth.

SEEK SUPPORT

As I mentioned in previous chapters, connecting with people who are supportive is essential to a successful recovery. You can connect with other people who are in recovery in free/donation-based support groups like AA, Buddhist recovery groups like Recovery Dharma, and CBT-based support groups like SMART Recovery. If you prefer a more mental health–focused support group, there are many groups available that are led by psychotherapists, which you can find on therapist directory sites like Psychology Today, Therapy Den, and Good Therapy.

In addition to group support, you may want to consider seeking the support of an individual therapist. You can find a therapist using the directories listed in the previous paragraph as well as through Inclusive Therapist, Zen Care, Network Therapy, and many more. If you want to use your insurance, you can search for a therapist who takes your insurance on the directories that I mentioned, or your insurance company probably has a list of therapists who are in network. If you have a PPO plan, most therapists will provide a receipt that you can use for potential reimbursement from your insurance company for a portion of the fee. If you don't have insurance and are in need of a low-fee therapist, you can try Open Path, a directory of therapists that provide low-fee therapy. If you have government-funded insurance, you can connect with your county services to find a therapist.

In the Moment

Put on some upbeat music that you like and dance vigorously. Let go of any embarrassment or inhibitions you may have. Nobody's watching! Shake your entire body. Shake your arms. Shake your legs. Make circles and figure eights with your hips. Jump up and down. After a few minutes of this, pause, take a few deep breaths, and sigh it out the mouth. Notice how you feel now. This is a great exercise to release tension, anxiety, and stress.

DEBRIEF AND DIGEST

In this chapter, we covered five key lessons:

- Mindfulness practices such as deep relaxation, progressive muscle relaxation, and visualization can help you relax and focus on your well-being rather than on alcohol.
- In order to make the switch to focusing on your wellness, it's necessary to examine and create new daily habits and practices that improve the quality of your sleep, nourishment, exercise habits, and relationships.
- Having a plan to deal with emotional, environmental, and social triggers when they occur will help you feel prepared and in control.
- Some strategies that you can use to support your sobriety and fuel your growth are starting a journal, avoiding social functions that involve alcohol, focusing on joyful movement, being mindful of your social media use, and developing a regular mindfulness practice.
- In addition to group support, there are many directories available to help you find the support of an individual therapist.

SELF CHECK-IN

Take a moment to reflect on how you feel. What emotions do you notice now that you have read and completed the exercises in this chapter? Where are you feeling them in your body and what do they feel like (color, texture, temperature, etc.)?

Take a moment to reflect on what you have learned in this chapter. What do you think will be the most helpful information to support your recovery?

_____

_____

_____

_____

_____

CLOSING: CONTINUE MOVING FORWARD

Congratulations! You made it to the end! Reading through a book like this and completing the exercises is not an easy thing to do. It required a great deal of courage, determination, and self-reflection, which is likely quite difficult for anyone in the throes of alcohol dependence. Consider doing something special for yourself to celebrate completing this workbook, like going out for a nice dinner, taking a warm bath, or getting a massage. You've earned it!

You've completed this important step, but your journey doesn't end here. There is so much more to come! Recovery is an ongoing practice, but with all the new skills you have learned and resources that you have become aware of, you can start to live a life that isn't dominated by an unhelpful relationship with alcohol. Many people tend to feel trapped and hopeless when they are in the chains of addiction, but sobriety can change all of that for the better. For many, sobriety has been the pathway to greater freedom and success as well as strengthened relationships with ourselves and others. My wish for you is that you get to experience all the benefits that a successful recovery has to offer.

RESOURCES

The following is a list of resources that includes books, recovery communities, and mindfulness apps that will encourage your self-motivation.

BOOKS

365 Ways to Have Fun Sober by Lisa M. Hann

AA Not the Only Way: Your One Stop Resource Guide to 12-Step Alternatives by Melanie Solomon

Alcoholics Anonymous, Fourth Edition: The Official "Big Book" from Alcoholics Anonymous by Alcoholics Anonymous World Services Inc.

Cognitive Behavioral Therapy Made Simple: 10 Strategies for Managing Anxiety, Depression, Anger, Panic, and Worry by Seth J. Gillihan, PhD

Her Best-Kept Secret: Why Women Drink—and How They Can Regain Control by Gabrielle Glaser

Inside Rehab: The Surprising Truth about Addiction Treatment—and How to Get Help That Works by Anne M. Fletcher

In the Realm of Hungry Ghosts: Close Encounters with Addiction by Gabor Maté, MD and Peter A. Levine

Powerless No Longer: Reprogramming Your Addictive Behavior by Peter W. Soderman

Quit Like a Woman: The Radical Choice to Not Drink in a Culture Obsessed with Alcohol by Holly Whitaker

Recover!: Stop Thinking Like an Addict and Reclaim Your Life by Stanton Peele and Ilse Thompson

Recovery Dharma: How to Use Buddhist Practices and Principles to Heal the Suffering of Addiction by Recovery Dharma

Recovery Options: The Complete Guide by Joseph Volpicelli, MD, PhD

Sex, Drugs, Gambling and Chocolate: A Workbook for Overcoming Addictions by A. Thomas Horvath, PhD

The Small Book: A Revolutionary Alternative for Overcoming Alcohol and Drug Dependence (Rational Recovery Systems) by Jack Trimpey, LCSW

SMART Recovery Handbook: Tools and Strategies to Help You on Your Recovery Journey by SMART Recovery and Rosemary Hardin

Sober for Good: New Solutions for Drinking Problems—Advice from Those Who Have Succeeded by Anne Fletcher, MS, RD

RECOVERY COMMUNITIES

Alcoholics Anonymous (AA.org)

Buddhist Recovery Program (RecoveryDharma.org)

In the Rooms (InTheRooms.com)

SMART Recovery (SmartRecovery.org)

MINDFULNESS APPS

Calm (Calm.com)

Headspace (Headspace.com)

Insight Timer (InsightTimer.com)

Waking Up (WakingUp.com)

REFERENCES

"5 Physical Benefits of Quitting Alcohol." Herren Wellness. January 31, 2019.
HerrenWellness.com/5-physical-benefits-of-quitting-alcohol.

Akbar, Mohammed, Mark Egli, Young-Eun Cho, Byoung-Joon Song, and Antonio Noronha.
"Medications for Alcohol Use Disorders: An Overview." *Pharmacology & Therapeutics*
185 (May 2018): 64–85. doi:10.1016/j.pharmthera.2017.11.007.

"Alcohol." Drugs.com. Accessed November 14, 2021. Drugs.com/alcohol.html.

"Alcohol and Blood Sugar." The Recovery Village Drug and Alcohol Rehab. Last modified
June 2, 2021. TheRecoveryVillage.com/alcohol-abuse/alcohol-and-blood-sugar.

"Alcohol and Depression." University at Buffalo Research Institute on Addictions.
November 13, 2018. Buffalo.edu/cria/news_events/es/es18.html.

"Alcohol Facts and Statistics." National Institute on Alcohol Abuse and Alcoholism.
Accessed November 16, 2021. NIAAA.NIH.gov/publications/brochures-and
-fact-sheets/alcohol-facts-and-statistics.

"Alcohol In Popular Culture." Alcohol Rehab Guide. Last modified October 15, 2021.
AlcoholRehabGuide.org/alcohol/alcohol-in-popular-culture.

"Alcohol Metabolism: An Update." National Institute on Alcohol Abuse and Alcoholism.
Accessed November 2, 2021. Pubs.NIAAA.NIH.gov/publications/aa72/aa72.htm.

"Alcohol Use and Your Health." Centers for Disease Control and Prevention. May 11, 2021.
CDC.gov/alcohol/fact-sheets/alcohol-use.htm.

"Alcohol Use Disorder: A Comparison between DSM-IV and DSM-5." National Institute
on Alcohol Abuse and Alcoholism. Accessed November 16, 2021. NIAAA.NIH.gov
/publications/brochures-and-fact-sheets/alcohol-use-disorder-comparison
-between-dsm.

"Alcohol's Damaging Effects on the Brain." National Institute on Alcohol Abuse and
Alcoholism. Accessed November 15, 2021. Pubs.NIAAA.NIH.gov/publications/aa63
/aa63.htm.

"Alcohol's Effects on the Body." National Institute on Alcohol Abuse and Alcoholism.
Accessed November 15, 2021. NIAAA.NIH.gov/alcohols-effects-health/alcohols
-effects-body.

Atigari, Onome V., Anne-Marie Kelly, Qamar Jabeen, and David Healy. "New Onset Alcohol Dependence Linked to Treatment with Selective Serotonin Reuptake Inhibitors." *The International Journal of Risk & Safety in Medicine* 25, no. 2 (2013): 105-9. doi:10.3233/JRS-130586.

Banerjee, Niladri. "Neurotransmitters in Alcoholism: A Review of Neurobiological and Genetic Studies." *Indian Journal of Human Genetics* 20, no. 1 (January 2014): 20-31. PubMed.NCBI.NLM.NIH.gov/24959010.

Brache, Kristina. "Advancing Interpersonal Therapy for Substance Use Disorders." *The American Journal of Drug and Alcohol Abuse* 38, no. 4 (2012): 293-98. doi:0.3109 /00952990.2011.643995.

Brookie, Kate L., Georgia I. Best, and Tamlin S. Conner. "Intake of Raw Fruits and Vegetables Is Associated with Better Mental Health than Intake of Processed Fruits and Vegetables." Frontiers. April 10, 2018. FrontiersIn.org/articles/10.3389/fpsyg.2018.00487/full.

Brookwell, Louise, Carys Hogan, David Healy, and Derelie Mangin. "Ninety-Three Cases of Alcohol Dependence Following SSRI Treatment." *International Journal of Risk & Safety in Medicine* 26, no. 2 (2014): 99-107. doi:10.3233/JRS-140616.

"Cognitive Distortions: Overgeneralizing." Cognitive Behavioral Therapy Los Angeles. July 21, 2016. CogBTherapy.com/cbt-blog/cognitive-distortions-overgeneralizing.

Di Chiara, Gaetano. "Alcohol and Dopamine." *Alcohol Health and Research World* 21, no. 2 (1997): 108-14. NCBI.NLM.NIH.gov/pmc/articles/PMC6826820.

"The Feminisation of Alcohol Marketing." BBC Worklife. Accessed November 13, 2021. BBC.com/worklife/article/20200924-the-feminisation-of-alcohol-marketing.

Fraga, Juli. "7 Physical Symptoms That Prove Depression Is Not Just 'In Your Head.'" Healthline. Last modified August 15, 2019. Healthline.com/health/mental-health /physical-symptoms-of-depression.

Germer, Christopher K., Ronald D. Siegel, Paul R. Fulton, and Andrew Olendzki. "The Roots of Mindfulness." In *Mindfulness and Psychotherapy*. New York: Guilford Press, 2016.

Gimeno, Carmen, Marisa Luisa Dorado, Carlos Roncero, Nestor Szerman, Pablo Vega, Vicent Balanzá-Martínez, and F. Javier Alvarez. "Treatment of Comorbid Alcohol Dependence and Anxiety Disorder: Review of the Scientific Evidence and Recommendations for Treatment." *Frontiers in Psychiatry* 8 (2017): 173. doi:10.3389 /fpsyt.2017.00173.

Głąbska, Dominika, Dominika Guzek, Barbara Groele, and Krystyna Gutkowska. "Fruit and Vegetable Intake and Mental Health in Adults: A Systematic Review." *Nutrients* 12, no. 1 (January 2020): 115. doi:10.3390/nu12010115.

Gorka, Stephanie M., Bina Ali, and Stacey B. Daughters. "The Role of Distress Tolerance in the Relationship between Depressive Symptoms and Problematic Alcohol Use." *Psychology of Addictive Behaviors* 26, no. 3 (2012): 621–26. doi:10.1037/a0026386.

"Gout." Centers for Disease Control and Prevention. July 27, 2020. CDC.gov/arthritis/basics/gout.html.

"Hangovers." National Institute on Alcohol Abuse and Alcoholism. Accessed November 16, 2021. NIAAA.NIH.gov/publications/brochures-and-fact-sheets/hangovers.

Hauser, Marion Boomer, and Frank Lynn Iber. "Nutritional Advice and Diet Instruction in Alcoholism Treatment." *Alcohol Health and Research World* 13, no. 3 (1988): 261. Link.Gale.com/apps/doc/A8193396/AONE?u=anon~701c8322&sid=googleScholar&xid=4ca965a4.

Healthwise Staff. "Stress Management: Doing Progressive Muscle Relaxation." University of Michigan Health. Accessed November 17, 2021. UofMhealth.org/health-library/uz2225.

Hirsch, Alex. "5 Major Sleep Disorders." SC Internal Medicine Associates & Rehabilitation. February 27, 2020. SCInternalMedicine.com/2020/02/28/5-major-sleep-disorders.

"Holiday Binge Drinking: Statistics & Data." American Addiction Centers. Accessed November 17, 2021. Alcohol.org/statistics-information/holiday-binge-drinking.

"How Much Physical Activity Do Adults Need?" Centers for Disease Control and Prevention. October 7, 2020. CDC.gov/physicalactivity/basics/adults/index.htm.

"Interpersonal Psychotherapy (IPT)." CAMH. Accessed November 16, 2021. CAMH.ca/en/health-info/mental-illness-and-addiction-index/interpersonal-psychotherapy.

"Is Alcohol Harming Your Stomach?" Drinkaware. Accessed November 2, 2021. Drinkaware.co.uk/facts/health-effects-of-alcohol/effects-on-the-body/is-alcohol-harming-your-stomach.

Jewell, Tim. "Does Alcohol Dehydrate You?" Healthline. May 23, 2019. Healthline.com/health/does-alcohol-dehydrate-you.

Johnston, Lloyd D., Richard A. Miech, Patrick M. O'Malley, Jerald G. Bachman, John E. Schulenberg, Megan E. Patrick, Michigan University Institute for Social Research. *Demographic Subgroup Trends among Adolescents in the Use of Various Licit and Illicit Drugs, 1975-2019.* (Monitoring the Future Occasional Paper Series. Paper 94). Ann Arbor, MI: Institute for Social Research, The University of Michigan, 2020. ERIC. ed.gov/?id=ED608241.

Kaskutas, Lee Ann. "Alcoholics Anonymous Effectiveness: Faith Meets Science." *Journal of Addictive Diseases* 28, no. 2 (2009): 145–57. doi:10.1080/10550880902772464.

Kay, Isa. "Is Your Mood Disorder a Symptom of Unstable Blood Sugar?" University of Michigan School of Public Health. October 21, 2019. SPH.UMich.edu/pursuit /2019posts/mood-blood-sugar-kujawski.html.

Kc, Ranjan, Robin Voigt, Xin Li, Christopher B. Forsyth, Michael B. Ellman, Keith C. Summa, Fred W. Turek, Ali Keshavarzian, Jae-Sung Kim, and Hee-Jeong Im. "Induction of Osteoarthritis-like Pathologic Changes by Chronic Alcohol Consumption in an Experimental Mouse Model." *Arthritis & Rheumatology* 67, no. 6 (June 2015): 1678–80. doi:10.1002/art.39090.

Kearney, David J., Carol A. Malte, Carolyn McManus, Michelle E. Martinez, Ben Felleman, and Tracy L. Simpson. "Loving-Kindness Meditation for Posttraumatic Stress Disorder: A Pilot Study." *Journal of Traumatic Stress* 26, no. 4 (August 2013): 426–34. doi:10.1002/jts.21832.

Krans, Brian. "Just the Taste of Beer Triggers a Dopamine Response in the Brain." Healthline. Last modified September 2, 2014. Healthline.com/health-news/mental -just-the-taste-of-alcohol-induces-a-craving-for-more-041613.

Littrell, Jill. "The Mind-Body Connection." *Social Work in Health Care* 46, no. 4 (2008): 17–37. doi:10.1300/j010v46n04_02.

Lovinger, David M. "Serotonin's Role in Alcohol's Effects on the Brain." *Alcohol Health and Research World* 21, no. 2 (1997): 114-20. NCBI.NLM.NIH.gov/pmc/articles /PMC6826824.

Manthey, Jakob, Kevin D. Shield, Margaret Rylett, Omer S. M. Hasan, Charlotte Probst, and Jürgen Rehm. "Global Alcohol Exposure between 1990 and 2017 and Forecasts until 2030: A Modelling Study." *The Lancet* 393, no. 10190 (June 2019): 2493–502. doi:10.1016/S0140-6736(18)32744-2.

Martin, Ryan. "What Is Overgeneralizing?" Psychology Today. Accessed November 17, 2021. PsychologyToday.com/us/blog/all-the-rage/201908/what-is-overgeneralizing.

Mayfield, R. D., R. A. Harris, and M. A. Schuckit. "Genetic Factors Influencing Alcohol Dependence." *British Journal of Pharmacology* 154, no. 2 (May 2008): 275–87. doi:10.1038 /bjp.2008.88.

McCann, Victoria. "Alcohol and Chest Pain: Causes, Symptoms" Castle Craig (blog). June 19, 2019. CastleCraig.co.uk/blog/2019/06/19/alcohol-chest-pain.

McDowell, April. "Short-Term Meditation Linked to Increased Blood Flow in the Brain, Increased Attention, and Better Self-Regulation." PsyPost. July 1, 2015. PsyPost .org/2015/07/short-term-meditation-linked-to-increased-blood-flow-in-the-brain -increased-attention-and-better-self-regulation-35395.

"Medication for Treating Anxiety Disorders in People with Alcohol Use Problems."
Cochrane. Accessed November 17, 2021. Cochrane.org/CD007505/DEPRESSN
_medication-treating-anxiety-disorders-people-alcohol-use-problems.

Narasimhan, Lakshmi, R. Nagarathna, and H. R. Nagendra. "Effect of Integrated Yogic
Practices on Positive and Negative Emotions in Healthy Adults." *International Journal
of Yoga* 4, no. 1 (2011): 13-19. doi:10.4103/0973-6131.78174.

Perney, Pascal, and Philippe Lehert. "Insomnia in Alcohol-Dependent Patients: Prevalence,
Risk Factors and Acamprosate Effect: An Individual Patient Data Meta-Analysis."
Alcohol and Alcoholism 53, no. 5 (September 2018): 611-18. doi:10.1093
/alcalc/agy013.

Pietrangelo, Ann. "Night Sweats and Alcohol." Healthline. Last modified February 5, 2021.
Healthline.com/health/night-sweats-and-alcohol#alcohol-night-sweats.

Raypole, Crystal. "How to Break a Habit (and Make It Stick)." Healthline. October 29, 2019.
Healthline.com/health/how-to-break-a-habit#reward-yourself.

Raypole, Crystal. "Why You Feel Depressed after Drinking and How to Handle It."
Healthline. July 30, 2020. Healthline.com/health/mental-health/depression
-after-drinking#takeaway.

"Risks: Alcohol Misuse." NHS. Accessed November 16, 2021. NHS.uk/conditions
/alcohol-misuse/risks/.

Roessler, Kirsten Kaya. "Exercise Treatment for Drug Abuse: A Danish Pilot Study."
Scandinavian Journal of Public Health 38, no. 6 (2010): 664-69. doi:10.1177
/1403494810371249.

Rutledge, Thomas. "How Meditation Improves Emotional and Physical Health." Psychology
Today. Accessed November 17, 2021. PsychologyToday.com/us/blog/the-healthy
-journey/201908/how-meditation-improves-emotional-and-physical-health.

Sánchez-Villegas, Almudena, Estefania Toledo, Jokin de Irala, Miguel Ruiz-Canela, Jorge
Pla-Vidal, and Miguel A. Martínez-González. "Fast-Food and Commercial Baked Goods
Consumption and the Risk of Depression." *Public Health Nutrition* 15, no. 3 (2011):
424-32. doi:10.1017/S1368980011001856.

Sayette, Michael A., Kasey G. Creswell, John D. Dimoff, Catharine E. Fairbairn, Jeffrey F.
Cohn, Bryan W. Heckman, Thomas R. Kirchner, John M. Levine, and Richard L. More-
land. "Alcohol and Group Formation: A Multimodal Investigation of the Effects of
Alcohol on Emotion and Social Bonding." *Psychological Science* 23, no. 8 (2012):
869-78. doi:10.1177/0956797611435134.

Scaccia, Annamarya. "Serotonin: What You Need to Know." Healthline. August 19, 2020. Healthline.com/health/mental-health/serotonin.

Scharff, Constance. "Neuroplasticity and Addiction Recovery." Psychology Today. Accessed November 17, 2021. PsychologyToday.com/us/blog/ending-addiction-good/201302 /neuroplasticity-and-addiction-recovery.

"Self-Compassion Guided Practices and Exercises." Self-Compassion.org. Accessed November 10, 2021. Self-Compassion.org/category/exercises/#.

Seltzer, Leon F. "You Only Get More of What You Resist—Why?" Psychology Today. Accessed November 17, 2021. PsychologyToday.com/us/blog/evolution-the-self/201606/you -only-get-more-what-you-resist-why.

Sharp, Rick L. "Role of Whole Foods in Promoting Hydration after Exercise in Humans." *Journal of the American College of Nutrition* 26, suppl. 5 (2007): 5925–65. doi:10 .1080/07315724.2007.10719664.

Siegel, Michael, Renee M. Johnson, Keshav Tyagi, Kathryn Power, Mark C. Lohsen, Amanda J. Ayers, and David H. Jernigan. "Alcohol Brand References in U.S. Popular Music, 2009–2011." *Substance Use & Misuse* 48, no. 13 (December 2013): 1475–84. doi:10 .3109/10826084.2013.793716.

"Sleep Disorders." NAMI. Accessed November 17, 2021. NAMI.org/About-Mental-Illness /Common-with-Mental-Illness/Sleep-Disorders.

Smith, Sara. "5-4-3-2-1 Coping Technique for Anxiety." University of Rochester Medical Center. Accessed November 18, 2021. URMC.Rochester.edu/behavioral-health -partners/bhp-blog/april-2018/5-4-3-2-1-coping-technique-for-anxiety.aspx.

Stanborough, Rebecca Joy. "How Black and White Thinking Hurts You (and What You Can Do to Change It)." Healthline. January 13, 2020. Healthline.com/health/mental-health /black-and-white-thinking.

Substance Abuse and Mental Health Services Administration. *Key Substance Use and Mental Health Indicators in the United States: Results from the 2019 National Survey on Drug Use and Health*. Rockville, MD: Center for Behavioral Health Statistics and Quality, Substance Abuse and Mental Health Services Administration, 2020. SAMHSA.gov /data/release/2019-national-survey-drug-use-and-health-nsduh-releases.

Suttie, Jill. "5 Science-Backed Reasons Mindfulness Meditation Is Good for Your Health." Mindful. October 29, 2018. Mindful.org/five-ways-mindfulness-meditation-is -good-for-your-health.

"Tips for Better Sleep." Centers for Disease Control and Prevention. July 15, 2016. CDC.gov/sleep/about_sleep/sleep_hygiene.html.

"Understanding the Dangers of Alcohol Overdose." National Institute on Alcohol Abuse and Alcoholism. Accessed November 16, 2021. NIAAA.NIH.gov/publications/brochures-and-fact-sheets/understanding-dangers-of-alcohol-overdose.

"Understanding the Stress Response." Harvard Health Publishing. July 6, 2020. Health.Harvard.edu/staying-healthy/understanding-the-stress-response.

Valentine, Matt. "3 CBT Techniques to Revisit Whenever You're Feeling Overwhelmed." Goalcast. Last modified September 5, 2019. Goalcast.com/cognitive-behavioral-therapy-to-succeed.

Volkow, Nora D., Gene-Jack Wang, Joanna S. Fowler, Dardo Tomasi, and Frank Telang. "Addiction: Beyond Dopamine Reward Circuitry." *Proceedings of the National Academy of Sciences of the United States of America* 108, no. 37 (September 2011): 15037–42. doi:10.1073/pnas.1010654108.

Volkow, Nora D., Roy A. Wise, and Ruben Baler. "The Dopamine Motive System: Implications for Drug and Food Addiction." *Nature Reviews Neuroscience* 18 (2017): 741–52. doi:10.1038/nrn.2017.130.

Watt, Anthony. "How Does Light Therapy Help Treat Depression?" Healthline. October 28, 2021. Healthline.com/health/depression/light-therapy#pros.

Welch, Ashley. "For a Longer Life, Researchers Say Eat This Many Fruits and Veggies per Day." CBS News. February 27, 2017. CBSnews.com/news/for-a-longer-life-researchers-say-eat-this-many-fruits-and-veggies-per-day.

"What Is the Endocrine System?" United States Environmental Protection Agency. Accessed November 16, 2021. EPA.gov/endocrine-disruption/what-endocrine-system.

Yao, Xiaoxin I., Michael Y. Ni, Felix Cheung, Joseph T. Wu, C. Mary Schooling, Gabriel M. Leung, and Herbert Pang. "Change in Moderate Alcohol Consumption and Quality of Life: Evidence from 2 Population-Based Cohorts." *Canadian Medical Association Journal* 191, no. 27 (July 2019): E753–60. doi:10.1503/cmaj.181583.

INDEX

curiosity about, 75
expressing, 81, 82
managing with alcohol, 5
physical sensations of, 18, 23
running away from, 73
sharing, 78, 134
sobriety benefits to, 115
tracking, 31
triggers, 36-37, 41, 137
uncomfortable, 89
Friendships, 112-113, 119

G
Gastritis, 19
Goal setting, 40-41, 114, 135
Gratitude, 90, 108
Grounding exercise, 82
Growth, 134-135, 137-138
Guided imagery, 127

H
Habits, 116-118, 140
Hands on heart meditation, 75
Hangovers, 18-19
Headaches, 18
Help, asking for, 9
Hope, 100-101, 121-122
Hormones, 27

I
"I feel" statements, 79
Interpersonal therapy (IPT), 51

J
Joint pain, 19
Journaling, 66, 68, 78, 137
Jumping to conclusions, 62-64
Jung, Carl, 73-74

L
Letting go, 102-103
LifeRing Secular Recovery, 52
Lifestyle changes, 114
Lightheadedness, 18

Limiting beliefs, 48. *See also*
Cognitive distortions
Littrell, Jill, 20

M
Major depressive disorder
(MDD), 52-53
Marketing. *See* Advertising
and marketing
Medications, 52-53
Meditation, 50-51, 75, 121
Mental health disorders, 12
Mindfulness practices,
20-22, 23, 50-51, 77 78,
126-127, 138, 140
Moderation, 118, 120
Monkey mind, 51
Movement, 21, 131-133,
138, 139
Muscle relaxation, 127

N
National Survey on Drug
Use and Health
(NSDUH), 6
Nausea, 19
Neuroplasticity, 116
Neurotransmitters, 26-28
Norepinephrine, 28

O
Overgeneralizing, 61-62
Overwhelm, 32, 40,
53, 68, 76, 82

P
Peer pressure, 4, 12
People-pleasing
behaviors, 4, 133
Planning ahead, 120, 123
Portion control, 37
Positive thinking, 88-90, 94
Progressive muscle
relaxation, 127

R
Radical acceptance, 72
Recovery Dharma, 41,
52, 100, 139
Recovery programs, 41,
51-52, 54, 100-101,
121-122, 139
Reframing, 58
Relationships, 133-134.
See also Friendships
Relaxation, 126-127
Risk factors for alcoholism,
11-12, 15
Rituals, 29-30, 32

S
Selective serotonin
reuptake inhibitors
(SSRIs), 52-53
Self-awareness, 35, 41
Self-compassion, 22, 54, 74
Self-esteem, 91-93, 94
Self-forgiveness, 86-88,
93, 121-122
Self-love, 53, 90
Self-talk, 89, 122
Self-worth, 92
Serotonin, 26-27, 28, 32
Sleep, 128-130
SMART Recovery, 41,
52, 100
Sobriety
benefits of, 115
challenges, 136-137
and social life, 120-122
stigma of, 106
Social drinking, 4-5,
7, 36-37
Social events and gatherings,
37, 112-113, 137
Social media, 138
Socioeconomic status, 7
Stigmas, 105-107, 108

ACKNOWLEDGMENTS

I'd like to acknowledge all my teachers, clinical supervisors, yoga instructors, clients, and loved ones for giving me the knowledge and support to complete this book.

ABOUT THE AUTHOR

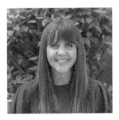 **Jennifer Leupp, LCSW,** is a licensed psychotherapist and yoga instructor in California. She specializes in working with women who struggle with substance abuse, trauma, and relationship challenges such as codependency utilizing EMDR (eye movement desensitization and reprocessing). Jeni also uses somatic and cognitive approaches and mindfulness to empower her clients to grow and heal. When she is not supporting clients, Jeni enjoys practicing yoga, singing, and going to the beach.

CPSIA information can be obtained
at www.ICGtesting.com
Printed in the USA
JSHW010931280322
24328JS00003B/3

9 781638 782971

SUCCESSFUL STRATEGIES *for* SOBER LIVING

Changing your relationship with alcohol is no small feat—but with the right tools you can curb your drinking habit and thrive. *Sobriety Workbook for Women* supports your journey to sober living, providing a nonjudgmental space to explore your relationship with alcohol and take steps toward healing.

The Science Behind Drinking
Learn about how alcohol can affect the brain and the body, as well as the risk factors for alcoholism and the societal pressures that often drive women to drink.

Engaging Exercises
Cultivate greater awareness and understanding of what triggers your drinking through mindfulness exercises, self check-ins, and more.

Awesome Affirmations
Enjoy a dose of positivity and perspective with uplifting affirmations you can turn to when you need a boost.

JENNIFER LEUPP, LCSW, is a licensed psychotherapist and yoga instructor based in California. She specializes in working with women and treating issues surrounding substance abuse, as well as relationship challenges like codependency and trauma.

U.S. $16.99   CAN $22.99   RO
ISBN 978-1-63878-297-1
51699

9 781638 782971

WWW.ROCKRIDGEPRESS.COM